A Quick Gu
Easing Pain
in the Workplace &
Beyond

Shara Ogin

Copyright

Audio Lessons

To access the accompanying Feldenkrais "Awareness Through Movement®" audio lessons, please see:
http://tinyurl.com/ycd9evez

Acknowledgements

I would like to bring many thanks to those who helped me with the completion of this book.

It has been a budding lesson which I have learned over the years that I don't have to do it alone. Good help is there right when you need it. All you have to do is spread your wings of intention and inspiration. It takes a team to bring an idea to fruition. And through community so much more is possible.

A special thanks to

Editor:	Peter Weverka
Illustrations:	Kat Williams
Book Interior Design:	Eric Lam
Book Cover Design:	Ashley Laughlin
Special images:	My Beloved Husband Frank Kuehnel
Photographs:	Laurel Doremus, PT & Kim McKee, PT
Nutritional info:	Luminalight.com

Table of Contents

Introduction

Are you tired of that old pain in the neck? The ache in your back? Or the familiar pain that radiates down to your hand? Do you feel more fatigued at the end of the workday than you should?

Many people struggle at work with a sore neck, tight upper shoulders, and occasional lower back pain. They brush it off as no big deal. Many people think this pain is "normal"; some blame it on old age.

But why live a life in pain when you could live a life of vitality? We know that when people feel good, their productivity and happiness in the workplace increases.

For almost two decades, I have treated office-related overuse injuries. In my work as a Feldenkrais practitioner®, occupational therapist, and ergonomist, I have developed the ability to quickly determine the factors that contribute to pain states. I have discovered many techniques for alleviating and preventing pain. This book presents the wealth of my experience as a health practitioner. It suggests ways to treat pain and describes treatment modalities that have helped my clients lead pain-free lives at work and at home.

Occupational and physical therapy are excellent approaches to pain management, particularly in cases that are acute or of relatively short duration. Through such therapies, one can learn what causes pain and learn techniques for preventing pain. A knowledge of body mechanics, stretching, and exercise programs can help relieve pain. So can modalities such as electrical stimulation, ultrasound, heat, and cold. Many therapy clients respond well to these approaches, (especially when in combination with ergonomic adaptations, rest, and a healthy lifestyle). While other patients face stubborn, obstinate pain with the usual treatment regimens.

When pain becomes more chronic, it has a wider impact on all the cells of the nervous system. Movement patterns become more undifferentiated and synergistic. Joints become more rigid and contracted. The muscles and viscera of the body, which are normally engaged when fleeing or on the lookout for danger, become activated during normal day-to-day activities.

This book focuses on physical pain. It offers clear-cut pain-management and prevention strategies. Whether your pain is acute or chronic, this book offers quick-tip solutions to get you back on your feet again, feeling well and vibrant.

I consider myself a teacher, one who teaches people how to utilize their minds and bodies more efficiently. A therapist, friend, parent or teacher can show you how to sit, stand, and move in a bio-mechanically correct way, yet until the movements are subcorticalized — in other words, ingrained at a subconscious level — the changes will be very short lived.

My mode of preference for this motor re-learning is called Feldenkrais. This method is named after Moshé Feldenkrais (1904-1984), a Ukranian-born scientist and judo master who founded it. He developed the method while rehabilitating from a recurring knee injury, in order to successfully avoid getting the surgery his doctors insisted he have.

The specific lessons I have chosen are all geared toward helping you to improve your ease and comfort when sitting for long periods of time in the workplace (and elsewhere). Some people report a lowering or decrease of their physical pain states after performing these lessons.

When performing the audio lessons (See accompanying CD or URL link on copyright pg of this book), please find a comfortable place to lie on a rug or carpet in a quiet space where you won't be interrupted for 35 minutes (approximately). Keep a small pillow or towel close by to support your head if needed. During the exercises one goal is to reduce muscular effort in order to increase your ability to feel.

In addition to somatic movement lessons this book offers:

- Low-cost solutions for how to set up your workstation.

- Tips to prevent the onset of repetitive strain injuries.

- Treatment suggestions for pain, swelling, eyestrain, and headaches

- Diet and fitness tips

Use this book as a guide to help you figure out what office equipment is right for you. Good equipment is not enough. I can't count the number of times I've seen people, with awkward postures and excessive effort, use top-of-the-line ergonomic chairs and keyboard equipment incorrectly.

After you become familiar with what a good fit feels like, you can adjust even the most basic office equipment to meet your needs. Office equipment should be fit to meet your needs, not the other way around. The equipment should be adapted to your body; your body shouldn't adapt to the equipment.

Over the past several years, the clients I treat for repetitive strain injuries have been getting progressively younger. In the social media and Silicon Valley companies I visit, it concerns me how individuals in the post-college age group carry themselves at their computers. They often hunch over their laptops with their heads rounded forward. Although most large companies have sufficient ergonomic programs, the individuals who work in these companies don't utilize the services — until they experience relentless pain.

Once pain begins, it is extremely difficult to stop. And once habits of poor usage become established, they are extremely difficult to break. That's why I encourage all my young clients to instill good postural habits from the start, before the pain sets in.

Treating office-related injuries can be easy if caught early enough and treated properly. Simply by correcting the workplace setup and adjusting the bio-mechanical use of your body, your pain and discomfort can readily be alleviated.

Take my hand and, together, let's stop the pain in its tracks!

1

The Pain Cycle for the Office Worker

During a workday, the typical office worker spends 7 to 7.5 hours in front of the computer. The office worker performs on average 10,000 to 15,000 keystrokes, or 1,730 keystrokes per hour. Sitting at a desk and tapping the keyboard takes its toll. By the end of the day, micro-tearing occurs in the fibers of the tendons, ligaments, and muscles.

Micro-tears are microscopic tears that occur in the connective tissues of the joints, tendons, and ligaments. Because these tears are so small, they don't result in any noticeable pain or constriction of movement — not at first, anyway. In a healthy individual, micro-tears repair themselves overnight. The ligaments and tendons are firm and strong by the time the office worker returns to work next day.

However, when muscles become overworked over a sustained period of time, a single night's rest may not be sufficient for the fibers to heal. An inflammatory response can result around the frayed fibers. This inflammation can impede the proper conduction of blood. It can pinch nerves and obstruct the flow of lymph, the fluid in the body's lymphatic system that contains infection-fighting white blood cells.

Eventually, overworked muscles start to fatigue, which has a negative effect on posture. You may find yourself hunched and rounded forward over your desk. As your back rounds and your head protrudes forward, the muscles on either side of your neck and spine have to work overtime to counterbalance this forward gravitational pull of the head. The ribs in front of the body become more compressed, constricting the organic flow of breath. Most office workers also perch forward in their chairs, which strains the stabilizing muscles of the lower back. These muscles have to work harder to keep the body erect and upright.

The result of all this is even more muscle fatigue. The office worker has to adjust his posture more frequently due to discomfort. Eventually he begins to utilize different, smaller, less-efficient muscle groups. Now muscles made for one purpose are being used for another, which can eventually lead to pain.

If the office worker is experiencing stresses from work, pressures from home, and other emotional difficulties, these contribute as well to his or her suboptimal posture.

The pain cycle has begun. This chapter takes a hard look at the pain cycle, how it progresses, and what its consequences are.

Compression of the Nerves

Besides slouching and bending over, an office worker when fatigued may put more weight on his elbows, forearms, and wrists. Too much sustained pressure on these parts of the body can potentially lead to a compression injury of the nerves, tendons, or arteries.

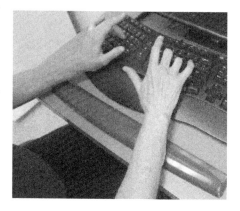

When nerves and tendons in the wrists are utilized repeatedly to type and move, especially in combination with poor postures and compression, this creates a double whammy. The person becomes even more susceptibility to injury.

Compression combined with movement of the wrists and hands puts the office worker in double jeopardy because friction is created where the tendons and soft tissues rub together. As soft tissues become irritated, they swell, which puts even more pressure on the underlying structures. The pinching, binding, or tugging around the nerves of these regions can inhibit nerve conduction. Delayed nerve conduction and impingement, in turn, can result in numbness, tingling, burning, and an aching sensation.

Pain Cycle

MusclesOverused

- Ligament & MM micro-tears
- Increased calcification
- Soft tissue impairments

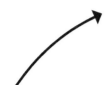

Difficulty Sleeping

- Decreased healing of micro tears & soft tissues

Postural Shifts

- Slouched sitting
- Rounded shoulders, head & neck
- Increased resting on elbows, forearms & wrists

Thalamus Alerted

- Pain suppressing hormones released
- Increased fear & anxiety

IncreasedDemandson

- Smaller muscle groups
- Tendons & nerves

ResistedTendonExcursion

- Muscles work harder

Decreased Circulation

- Less O2 supply & toxin removal
- Fluid accumulation

Injuries such as carpal tunnel syndrome can result where, the nerve that runs through the bones of the wrist (known as the carpal tunnel) becomes constricted. This results in the experience of tingling, burning, and numbness in the thumb and next two fingers as well as a weakness of the hand.

In order to contract, muscles require impulses from the nerves. When nerves are impinged, the signal they send to the muscles is weakened. This can directly impact the strength of a muscle. (This book describes some nerve-stretching exercises in the case you do have a nerve injury or are experiencing nerve symptoms.)

Compression combined with movement of the wrists and hands puts the office worker in double jeopardy because friction is created where the tendons and soft tissues rub together.

Sluggish Blood and Lymph Flow

Nerves aren't the only part of the body that is compressed when you slump at your desk or exhibit poor posture as you work. Like nerves, blood vessels travel through your wrists and elbows. When compressed, blood vessels also function less efficiently.

Blood has two main purposes. The first is to remove waste products such as carbon dioxide. The second is to deliver oxygen and other life-giving nutrients throughout the body, including hormones, temperature-regulating elements, minerals, and vitamins.

When blood flow is impeded, fewer waste products are removed and less oxygen is distributed to the body's extremities. This affects the proper functioning of the organs and muscles of your body.

Edema can be viewed as a red flag warning signal that something in your body is not functioning as efficiently or optimally as it should.

Lymph is one of the systems responsible for ridding your body of toxins and waste and delivering white blood cells to your body. White blood cells are essential for fighting infections.

Accumulation of waste as well as a malfunctioning lymphatic system can result in "pooling" or edema in the extremities of the body and around injury sites. In general, edema can be viewed as a red flag warning signal that something in your body is not functioning as efficiently or optimally as it should. Please note, however, that many conditions can cause inflammation. Pregnancy, arthritis, and even a solid night's sleep can cause your body to swell.

Stiff and Constrained Tendons

Bad posture at your desk also has a negative effect on tendons. Tendons connect muscles to bones. They are made of collagen, a strong, high-protein type of tissue. When a muscle contracts, the tendon goes into action. It pulls or pushes a bone according to instructions from the muscle.

Tendons typically glide back and forth through a very viscous and water-like fluid composed primarily of blood. However, when inflammation occurs near a tendon, the fluid through which the tendon moves thickens. This makes each glide of the tendon more difficult. The result is weakness and possibly a loss of motion.

As an analogy, imagine trying to swim through a pool of molasses rather than a pool of water. The added effort your body would experience while pushing through the molasses is equivalent to the extra effort the tendon must make when it encounters inflammation.

Another result of inflammation is that the sheath of the tendon may become inflamed. This can result in tenosynovitis (the swelling of the fluid-filled sheath called the synovium that surrounds the tendon) or tendonitis (the swelling of the tendon itself). Symptoms include pain, swelling of soft tissues, and difficulty moving the particular joint where the inflammation occurs.

When a tendon is compressed or when its movement requires maneuvering around a bent joint (or corner), more effort is required. As more "work" is required, distal or smaller, less efficient muscles are then recruited to take over more of the work.

Stiff and Restricted Muscles

The muscles in our bodies twist and weave around one another. Functionally speaking, no muscle is used in isolation. Rather, the fabric of communication from one muscle deeply influences the muscles above, below, and all around it. Hence, when one muscle is being over worked, so too are neighboring muscles, and the neighboring muscles will eventually begin to fatigue. Over time, trigger points and soft tissue tenderness can develop. (During Feldenkrais lessons it's really interesting to explore the subtle connection between various muscle groups and see to what degree you can isolate individual muscles)!

The muscles in our bodies twist and weave around one another

After an injury, the body's natural reaction is to guard and protect the area of injury. But when the body restricts movement in a particular region, structures around the injury site also become more restricted and static.

For example, consider someone who has a herniated disc at L4-5. The movements of the associated ligaments, tendons, muscles, and joints surrounding this region will also be compromised. In other words, the surrounding muscles will over time become more stiff and rigid.

Muscular "holding" is a natural protective reaction; it limits further injury or assault. After any tendon, muscle, bone, or joint injury, the protocol is always to limit motion so that healing can occur. If extreme immobilization is recommended — for example, after a muscle tear or bone fracture — a cast or firm static splint is applied.

> Muscular "holding" is a natural protective reaction; it limits further injury or assault.

Following the removal of the immobilization device, when movement is allowed, not only will the structures at the injury site be less pliable and mobile, but the uninvolved soft tissues and other structures around it will also lose their elasticity and mobility. When this occurs, it is customary for your body to begin to function in a less differentiated and integrated manner. The movements of the body in and around the region may become less coordinated and connected.

For example, if you have a right shoulder injury, the areas around the shoulder girdle may stiffen and contract. Over time, the right scapula may not glide as efficiently. The left scapula and shoulder complex may then compensate with even more movement (or less). This new motor pattern will affect the entire organization of other structures throughout your body, including your ribs, hips, and the lower extremities on both sides.

You may find differences in your gait with one leg or hip being stiffer. You may find one leg to be heavier, longer, and louder with each step. You may find when you sit that more weight is distributed on one sit bone than the other. You may find your ribs compressed on one side while lengthened on the other. This can affect your overall balance, stability and agility.

This is just one example of how the body organization shifts following an injury. Try contracting your right shoulder while walking and then see for yourself what sort of differences you notice.

Most computer users have their shoulder and upper trapezium muscles raised up, not only when they are working, but even at rest. This not only decreases the size of the "tunnel" where nerves, arteries, and lymph travel through to the arm, it also sets up an unconscious pattern of overworking muscles which would otherwise be resting.

Yet working long hours at your job doesn't have to hurt. With the correct workplace setup and the correct use of your body, your pain and discomfort can be alleviated.

Exercise:

Getting Acquainted with the Pain

One of the first steps to alleviating pain is getting to know it from the inside and out. We're accustomed to treating pain as "the enemy," but I invite you instead to treat it as a friend. After all, it is a part of us, welcome or not.

Begin to familiarize yourself with what this part of yourself — your pain — likes and dislikes most. What activities or times of day does it prefer and why? Who does it respond positively to, and who does it respond negatively to?

1. On a scale from 1 to 10, 0 being no pain and 10 meaning the pain that would send you to the hospital:
    *   What is your pain level now?
    *   What is your pain level typically when you wake up?
    *   What is your pain level at the end of the work day?
    *   What is your pain level at rest?
    *   What is your pain level when performing day to day tasks?

2. What aggravates your pain?

3. What eases your pain?

4. Is there anyone In your life who gives your emotional distress?
    *   If yes, how does your body react when triggered by that person?
    *   How does this affect the pain you feel?
    *   How would you rather feel around the person?
    *   What steps can you take to ensure this feeling in your body?

5. Is there any thing in your life that gives you emotional distress?

- If yes, how does your body react when triggered by it?
- How does this affect the pain in your body?
- How would you rather feel when around this emotional trigger?
- What steps can you take right now to better ensure this feeling in your body?

6. If your pain had a message, what might this message be?

By familiarizing ourselves with pain as if it were a friend rather than a foreign invader or enemy, you can start to better meet your pain's needs and give it the attention it deserves. Not the "poor me" sort of attention, but the attention of listening to what in the system is off and in need of balancing.

2

Ergonomics

―――――――

There are two ways to combat and prevent pain in the workplace. One is by changing the way you organize and so-to-speak use yourself. The other is to change the ergonomic design of the place where you do your work — in other words, to customize your workstation.

> There are two ways to combat and prevent pain the workplace.

I use the term "workstation" to apply to your desk, chair, and computer monitor, and other physical things that come into play when you do your work. A proper workstation set is crucial for the defense and prevention of musculoskeletal injuries. Even the most fit and healthy person is prone to getting pain when working in a station that is not ergonomically designed and set up to fit his or her body dimensions.

This chapter explains everything you need to know to set up a basic computer work station.

Everyone has different anthropometric measurements. Everyone has different-sized limbs, a different height and weight, and a different height to weight ratio. For that reason, no workstation setup can fit every individual. This is why adjustability is key! It is crucial to adjust the workplace to the height, width, dimensions and job tasks of the individual.

Learning How to Sit

As you read this, ask yourself this question and do your best to answer it honestly: How are you sitting? It's not a question people ask themselves very often, yet over half the average person's waking hours are spent sitting. It's not an easy question to answer.

To get specific answers to this all-important question, ask yourself these questions. They will help you understand how you sit:

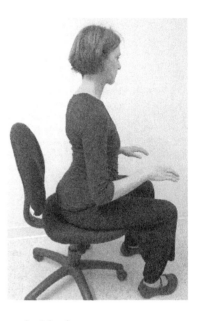

1. Is your head rounded or protruding forward? Or is your sitting more upright and erect?

2. Are you experiencing any low back or neck tightness and discomfort?

3. How is your breathing? What parts of yourself — your lungs, chest, throat, mouth — are breathing?

It is perfectly normal in this day and age to be unaware of your posture. Unfortunately, most people sit in ways that make their bodies work harder than they need to.

An office worker who perches forward toward the edge of the chair when performing a static repetitive task may appear to be sitting in a healthy position. The worker's back may look anatomically "straight." Very likely, however, the person is inhibiting his breath, particularly in the chest, and over contracts the muscles of the low back in order to stabilize the torso.

When you slouch, the lower back — one of the body's largest and strongest muscle groups — is put in a lengthened position. This restricts and limits the muscle's availability for movement.

Slouching vs. Upright Sitting

Consider what happens when you slouch as you sit. The medial inferior border of the shoulder blade (the scapula) "wings" away from the torso (thorax). This alters the angle of the entire shoulder complex. Meanwhile, the forward rounding of the head and neck requires excessive contraction of the posterior neck muscles to counterbalance the forward gravitational pull that occurs when the

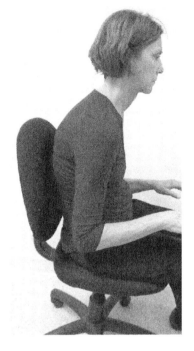

head and neck round forward. With slouched and rounded forward sitting, breathing becomes compromised. The muscles of the back become less available to assist with movement, which then results in more effort to raise and move the arm.

In optimal upright sitting, the vertebra of the spine stack one on top of another. Almost no muscular or active forces from ligaments are required and the amount of intervertebral pressure (pressure between each vertebra) and muscular effort throughout the torso is at a minimum.

In the spine, stacked from your head to your "tail," there are seven cervical vertebrae, twelve thoracic, seven lumbar, five fused sacral, and three to five fused coccyx vertebrae. You can see how the shape of the vertebral column actually forms an "S" shape. Like pieces of a puzzle, each vertebral bone is formed and shaped to snap perfectly in place one on top of the other.

In the course of day-to-day actions, this "S" changes shape. When your go to bat in a baseball game, pick up a pencil from the floor, or engage in most movements that require the entire body, the spine needs to bend, twist, and rotate according to the task it undertakes.

In optimal upright sitting, the verebra of the spine stack one on top of another.

When you're doing sustained and static work, maintaining a spine as close to the "S position as possible is crucial for your health and crucial to the most efficient use of your body. Keeping your spine in the "S" shape keeps the inter-vertebral pressure in an optimal state, which then assists with the following:

- More freedom of movement of the arms and hands

- Improved work endurance (as a result of less muscular fatigue)

- Longer periods of focus and comfort, as carrying the neck and head on the spine minimizes eye and neck fatigue

A typical slouched posture requires less muscular effort, which is why many people find more comfort in this position. In this position, however, more pressure is put on the front (or anterior) part of each

Sitting Exercise:

Finding a Good Sitting Balance

What is the happy medium between sitting bolt upright and slouching? Try this exercise to find the answer.

1. Sit up nice and tall in a chair with no back support.

2. Puff out your chest to mimic an upright military sitting posture. This may be your instinctual sitting posture when asked to sit tall. The position you are in now is an example of good intervertebral alignment and pressure, but it requires too much muscular effort to maintain. Notice how inhibited your breathing muscles are, particularly in your chest. Notice as well how much muscle contraction is occurring in your low back.

3. Try slouching, the opposite sitting posture. Allow your back to round and your pelvis to tilt back as your head roles slightly forward of your torso. What is happening here to your breath and the amount of muscular effort throughout your body?

4. Go back and forth between these two postures a few times to experience the difference between the two extremes. Feel your body roll back and forth between the back of your sit bones and the heads of the two sit bones.

5. Stop in the position between these two extremes, where you're sitting on the heads of your two sit bones. From here, scoot back in your chair so your lower back comes into contact with the lumbar support (lumbar support is explained in the next chapter).

Congratulations. You've now found your optimal sitting posture.

vertebra. Over time, this pushes the gelatinous fluid (which functions to cushion compressive forces of the spine) between each vertebra backwards. Eventually the fluid and intervertebral pressures can compromise nerves and arteries. The slouched posture also puts the articulating muscles at a disadvantaged state, requiring them to work harder.

Adjusting Your Chair

For optimal sitting, the S-shaped curve of the spine must be maintained.

For optimal sitting, the S-shaped curve of the spine must be maintained. Whenever the inward curve of the lower back is lessened or lost (and the back nears a "C" shape), or when the curve is overly pronounced forward as in a lordotic curve (pronounced inward curve of the five lumbar vertebrae), pressures and tensions build quickly. This can be a precursor to back, neck, and upper extremity problems.

It is crucial for the lumbar area of your back to be properly supported when you sit. Some chairs do not provide lumbar support. In some chairs the lumbar support is not in the optimal position. Most ergonomic chairs have adjustable lumbar supports so you can adjust the back support according to your needs.

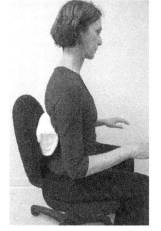

If your chair is not adjustable, you can improvise by adding an external lumbar support. A variety of external lumbar supports are available online and even in department stores. My favorite is the simple half lumbar roll secured with an adjustable strap. The problem with most external lumbar supports is that they can be difficult to keep in place; they tend to fall down to the seat pan under their own weight. You want the most pronounced part of the lumbar support to fit into the most inward curve of your back. For a quick fix, you can improvise with a small towel rolled up, taped together, and inserted into your lumbar region.

Supporting any area above your lumbar region against the back of your chair is unnecessary. Supporting the upper back only inhibits the glide of your shoulder blades. Your upper-back region should be free to assist with movements of the arms (such as typing or reaching forward for your mouse or phone).

Sitting Exercise:

Seated Stretching Exercise

Sitting at a desk, people frequently lean, reach, and round forward repeatedly in the same direction. For the sake of alignment, it is important to stretch in the opposite direction.

1.   If your chair has a back-tilt mechanism, unlock it.

2.   Lean back in your chair with your arms extending freely over your head.

3.   Let your back and neck relax into extension as you take two or three deep, full breaths. Make sure that the back tilt mechanism is locked when you resume working.

Other seated stretches include rotating to the right and rotating to the left. Hold each side for five to seven seconds while side-bending with one arm over your head (as will be demonstrated in the standing stretches below).

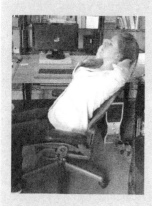 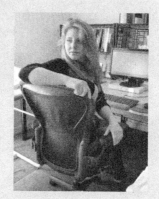

When the lower curves of your spine are supported in their neutral alignment, all the vertebrae stack one on top of the other in an upright, aligned posture, and your head is fully supported over your pelvis.

Here's a tip: If you have a tendency to slouch, you can make sure you're sitting on the heads of your pelvis by rolling up a small washcloth and positioning it just behind your two sit bones. This rolls your pelvis ever so slightly forward and helps position your pelvis in a more neutral alignment. It minimizes the amount of muscle effort and maximizes spinal alignment.

Finding Optimal Chair Height

The height of your chair is important. If your chair is too high, your heels can't rest solidly on the floor. This has several negative health consequences:

Pressure on the nerves and structures on the back of your thighs increase. This can compromise blood circulation and squeeze the nerves in your lower extremities.

The ground forces that are transmitted from the ground up through your feet to the rest of your body are affected. Maintaining a consistent ground force is crucial for optimal static and dynamic sitting.

Components of an Ergonomic Chair

An ergonomic chair ideally has the following five components:

- An adjustable seat height

- Light padding or cushioned seat

- An adjustable seat with a front waterfall edge (cushion that slopes gradually)

- No arm rests or removable armrests

- Lumbar support

After you have properly adjusted your chair, sit in it and scoot all the way back into your chair so the back of your pelvis touches the back of the chair. Your weight should be balanced between the heads of both sit bones. Your head should be over your pelvis. The lumbar support of the chair should fit like a lock and key into the small of your back.

Adjusting the Chair Armrests

Do you look like the person in the illustration when at work?

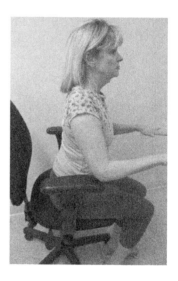

If you do, the first question to ask yourself is whether the armrests on your chair or desk are raised up too high. When armrests are too high, it results in you, too, raising your arms and shoulders when you're working. Over time, this can constrict the nerve flow that runs from your neck, down your arm. It can also inhibit the availability of movement of your shoulder blade and upper back region, making it so that your hands and arms need to take over more of the work that your proximal musculature would have done otherwise. Even when typing, using a mouse, and turning pages of documents, a significant amount of upper back and shoulder involvement is required.

I recommend lowering your armrests so they are below the height of your elbows and out of the way. In some cases, however, using arm rests can make you significantly more comfortable. Hunt and peck typists, people with severe arm pain, and individuals with larger builds seem to often find more comfort with resting their arms on armrests.

If you do use armrests, make sure they are in line with, or are slightly higher than, the height of the table or desk at which you work. By aligning your desk and armrests, you avoid hitting or resting on the sharp edge of the desk (which could result in compression injuries). Also, make sure there is a significant amount of padding on your chair armrest to minimize pressure on your elbows and forearms.

Most computer users have their shoulder and upper trapezium muscles raised up, not only when they work, but also at rest. Unless someone points it out or we're looking at ourselves in the mirror, most of us are completely unaware of how raised our shoulders are.

Raising the shoulders not only decreases the size of the "tunnel" through which nerves and arteries travel down to the arm, it also sets up an unconscious pattern of over firing or overworking in this region, despite the fact that no work is required. When a person habitually over contracts her upper trapezius, she also over contracts the neighboring muscles of the cervical spine.

Zones of Comfort

Ideally, you want to spend the majority of your workday using your arms primarily in what I call the "zone of comfort." In this zone, your body functions most efficiently and requires the least amount of effort to complete tasks. The zone of comfort is where you want your arms to function for as much of the workday as possible (with the exception of stretches and breaks, of course). Be sure to position your keyboard, mouse, and any other frequently used items in the zone of comfort.

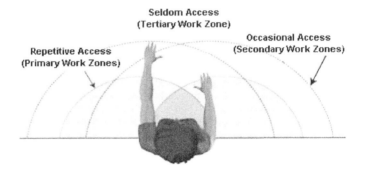

Follow these steps to find your zone of comfort:

1. Hold a full water bottle or a two-pound weight in one hand.

2. Bend your elbow to 90 degrees while holding the weight. Circle your arm in the area where you sense the most arm comfort. This is your zone of comfort.

3. Double the size of this circle. Feel how the weight of the item you are holding doubles or triples. Now you are operating outside your zone of comfort. This is the secondary zone where items should be accessed only occasionally.

4. Straighten your elbow and make a circle with the weight while maintaining the full length of your arm. Feel how the weight of this item feels like it has increased four to five times (if not

more). Notice as well that you can feel the pressure in your shoulder, neck, and upper back. This far zone — you could call it the zone of discomfort —should be accessed very seldom throughout the workday. Go here only when you have to reach for the phone or a similar item.

Whenever a task requires you to leave the zone of comfort, if possible stand or physically move your body to complete the task. Try to minimize the amount of arm reach. Maintaining good body mechanics means always working in your zone of comfort. Your sternum and belly button should face in the direction of your work. Minimize twisting and reaching while performing tasks. Strive to stay in your zone of comfort during 90 percent of your workday.

If your ergonomic setup or your job tasks require you to leave your zone of comfort often, take more frequent stretch breaks. Doing so counterbalances the excessive stress on your joints and muscles.

Workplace Stretches

For all Stretches stop before the point of pain.

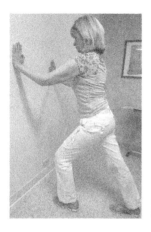

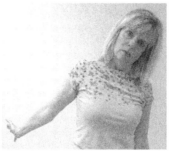

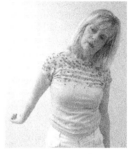

Quadricep stretch. Lean into front knee until you feel a sustained stretch (hold 5-7 sec.)

Wrist extended back, ear towards opposite shoulder (hold 5-7 sec. each side).

Wrist flexed, ear towards opposite shoulder (hold 5-7 sec. each side).

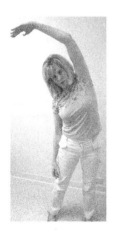

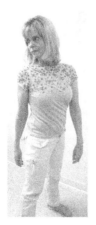

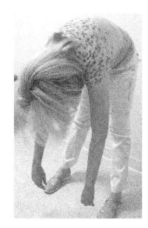

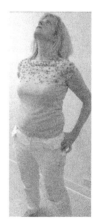

Side bend with arm over head (3 times each side).

Twist side to side (3 times each side).

Forward bend (hold 5-7 seconds). Come up slowly, vertebra by vertebra.

Back bend, hold 5-7 seconds.

Sitting Exercise:

Finding the Optimal Position of the Pelvis

Try this exercise to rest your upper shoulders:

1. Rest your arms and hands on your lap.

2. Inhale and very slowly raise one of your shoulders towards your ear, then exhale and allow your shoulder to relax gently back and down.

3. Repeat step 2 three or four more times slowly and smoothly (try it with your eyes closed). Each time you do this, allow your shoulder to lower just a little bit more.

4. Pause and notice if one shoulder feels lower than the other. If it doesn't, tightly contract that same shoulder up towards that ear and hold it tight, tighter, and even tighter for seven seconds. Then let it go completely.

5. This exercise is also great to do lying down on your back with a towel roll placed between your shoulder blades. Or while lying on a six-inch-thick foam roller.

Sitting Exercise:

Finding the Proper Height for Your Chair

To figure out the proper height of your chair, follow these steps.

1. With your feet, roll the chair forward and backwards, left and right several times. That's right, do a little chair dance.

2. Notice how much effort it takes from your legs to move the chair.

3. Lower the chair a small amount and do the same "chair dance." Is it easier or harder to move the chair from this height?

4. If it is easier, go a bit lower and repeat the same exercise. If it is harder, raise the chair a little above the point it was initially at.

5. Keep with this inquiry until you find the height that requires the least amount of effort to move the chair. The optimal height of your chair will have a 90-110 degree angle at your knees, or your hips will be just slightly higher than your knees.

Sitting Exercise:

Finding the Optimal Position of the Pelvis

To find your optimal sitting posture, perform this simple exercise

1. Sit towards the front half of your chair.

2. Notice whether your legs are close together or wide apart. It is recommended for women to keep their legs approximately hips-width apart; and men approximately shoulder-width apart. Experiment to find out which distance between your legs provides the most comfort and support.

3. Notice whether you are sitting more on one sit bone than on the other.

4. Gently roll your pelvis forward so your weight shifts to the front of your sit bones.

5. Gently roll your pelvis back so you feel the weight shift to the back of each sit bone. Do this several times. You may notice your head rising up as your pelvis rolls forward and lowering as you roll back.

6. Stop when you find the spot in the middle of these two extremes, where your weight is equally balanced between the two bony prominences known as your sit bones (your ischial tuberosities).

7. Gently rock your weight onto your right sit bone, then rock it to the left sit bone. Do this several times.

8. Stop in the middle so you are sitting more or less on the heads of both sit bones.

Congratulations. You have found the optimal position of your pelvis when seated for office work. Scoot back into your chair until you feel the back of your pelvis making contact with the back of your chair. Make sure the lumbar support of the chair fits directly into the small of your back. If you are uncertain where this is, touch your low back with the back of your hand and feel if the inward curve of the chair contacts you there.

3

Finding Comfort With the Keyboard and Mouse

Thus far the focus of this book has been on sitting. The next subject is how to work comfortably with your computer devices — namely with your keyboard and mouse. Since the majority of people spend their work day with these two devices, I decided to devote a chapter to using them optimally and comfortably.

Adjusting the Keyboard

The traditional keyboard has two mini "kickstands" or legs in the back and a numeric ten-key pad located on the right. Usually the mouse is positioned to the right of the keyboard, which often results in an excessive amount of right arm abduction to access the mouse.

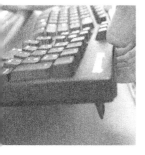

If you don't use your numeric ten-key pad and you're willing to alternatively use the number keys at the top of the keyboard, consider purchasing a "mini" keyboard or one without the 10-key pad. You can purchase a flat, mini-keyboard or a split keyboard such as the gold touch or kinesis. The split in the keyboard helps provide a neutral arm and hand position.

Keyboard Exercise:

Finding the Optimal Keyboard Split

Try this exercise to find a comfortable position for your keyboard.

1. Sitting comfortably in a chair with your upper arms relaxed, bend your elbows to 90 degrees. Have your thumbs facing up.

2. Very gently rotate your forearms so your palms face up toward the ceiling. As you do this, close your eyes and go very slowly so you can sense the amount of pull or stretch throughout your forearm.

3. Rotate your arms the opposite way so your palms face toward the floor. Feel the pull once again in this position.

4. Go back and forth a few times between the palms-up and palms-down position, and then stop in a comfortable position between the two extremes. In this position you feel the least amount of pull throughout your arm. This is where your muscles function most optimally.

5. Adjust the split of your keyboard to this angle (some people prefer to flatten the keyboard just a few degrees more than this angle).

If you do use the 10-key pad, consider altering the position of the mouse from the right to the left side of the keyboard from time to time, especially

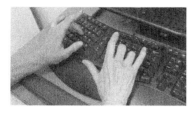

if you have right arm or hand pain. Computer operating systems all offer the ability to switch mouse hands. If you are a right-handed mouser, learning to maneuver the mouse with your left hand may take time, but the health benefits will be worth the trouble.

Most computer users habitually hyper-extend one or more fingers, actively engaging all the fingers unnecessarily. Only the fingers needed for the task should be actively engaged.

When certain fingers are consistently held in extension, the extensor muscles of the fingers and hand end up working overtime when they could otherwise be resting. This unconscious and unnecessary habit can result in tightness around the back of the forearm.

Long finger nails impede the ability to maintain a natural "C" shape of the fingers when typing. This is because the typist will find themselves straightening their fingers and adjusting their hand posture in order to type with the pads of each finger (as opposed to using their finger tips). Hence, putting excess and unnecessary work upon the extensor musculature (as discussed). Over time, this can result in pain up the back side of the arm, tightness in their shoulders and possibly even arthritic like conditions in the distal joints of the fingers.

The proper way to type is with the tip of each finger lightly stroking each key of the keyboard while maintaining a neutral and soft bend at all three joints of the fingers."

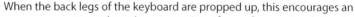

When the back legs of the keyboard are propped up, this encourages an

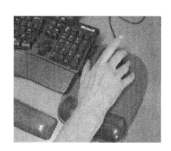

upward reach or extension of your fingers. A solution to this problem is to lower the back legs of the keyboard so the keyboard sits flat on the table. If you use a keyboard platform, you can angle it so the back of it is tilted downward as well. This is known as a "negative tilt" of the keyboard platform.

Learning the Proper Mouse

The most important thing to know about mousing is this: Fully drape your fingers over the top of the mouse buttons and completely relax the palm of your hand over the face of the mouse. In this position the natural arches of your hand and curves of your fingers are completely supported.

To find this neutral hand posture, simply drop your arms to your sides and notice the crescent or "C" shape your fingers naturally assume when they are at rest. Notice whether your wrist falls straight. This is your neutral finger and wrist position. Although it varies from person to person, a neutral wrist posture is from - 5 to -15 degrees.

Maintaining a neutral wrist posture is paramount. If your wrist is flexed as you work, the flexor muscle groups that bend your wrist and fingers forward shorten; the extensor muscle groups of the arm

The most important thing to know about mousing is this: Fully drape your fingers over the top of the mouse buttons and completely relax the palm of your hand over the face of the mouse. In this position the natural arches of your hand and curves of your fingers are completely supported.

To find this neutral hand posture, simply drop your arms to your sides and notice the crescent or "C" shape your fingers naturally assume when they are at rest. Notice whether your wrist falls straight. This is your neutral finger and wrist position. Although it varies from person to person, a neutral wrist posture is from - 5 to -15 degrees.

Maintaining a neutral wrist posture is paramount. If your wrist is flexed as you work, the flexor muscle groups that bend your wrist and fingers forward shorten; the extensor muscle groups of the arm that bend your wrist and fingers backward lengthen. The opposite is true when you work with your wrist in extension. Both extremes place your muscles in a weakened position and could, over time, result in nerve compression injuries and muscular pain.

When you mouse, you only really need to drop your fingers down to click the buttons, rather than reaching your fingers up or straight. Extending your fingers up to meet the keys or mouse button is an unconscious habit that most computer users are guilty of.

If the mouse is too small to fully support the concave shape of your hand, try using a larger and more contoured mouse. By "contoured" I mean a mouse that fits the natural curves and arches of your hand. A contoured mouse provides support under the index finger that is slightly higher than the support under the pinky.

For men or women with broad and open shoulders, a vertical mouse is ideal. This type of mouse prevents the inferior border of their shoulder blade from flaring off the mouse user's back.

4

Finding Comfort With Your Laptop

Looking down for sustained periods of time at a laptop monitor results in a great deal of neck flexion; eventually it can lead to posterior neck tightness and strain. Looking down at a laptop monitor may also compromise the posture of your arms if your shoulders and forearms are elevated to reach the keyboard.

If you work on a laptop continuously or for more than two to three total hours per day, get a laptop riser to elevate your screen and use an external mouse and keyboard. I highly recommend elevating the screen. As a low-cost option, you can use a large three-ring binder to raise your monitor or simply stack it on books.

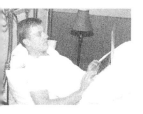

However, when the laptop is raised on a table or riser, your arms eventually can become overworked and fatigued. If you are like me and frequently use your laptop while lying in bed or on a couch, position your spine as straight as possible. Use two pillows to keep your upper back, neck, and head all inline. Above all, avoid the hyper-flexed neck posture. Use pillow support as necessary under your arms while maintaining a neutral wrist and fingers.

Head/Neck Exercise:

Finding a Neutral Posture

This exercise is designed to help you find a neutral head and neck posture when gazing at your monitor. Perform all the movements slowly while staying in your comfort range.

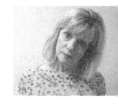

1. Close your eyes. Bring your right ear towards your right shoulder. Then bring your left ear towards your left shoulder. Repeat this three times. Then stop in the middle to rest

2. Notice whether your head and nose feel centered between your right and left shoulder. If not, bend your head a couple more time the opposite way. Then recheck.

3. Look up slowly. Look down slowly. Then repeat these movements three times, stopping in the middle to rest.

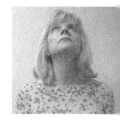

4. Notice whether your head and nose feel centered between the two extremes and your nose is along the horizon. If not, angle your head one more time the opposite way. Then recheck.

5. Turn your head to the right, and then to the left. Repeat these movements three times moving slowly. Come back to the middle and rest.

6. Notice how your head is balanced between these two extremes. If it's rotated more to one direction, slowly rotate your head two to three times to the opposite direction.

If you are uncertain if you've found your neutral head and neck postures, looking into the mirror between each step might be helpful.

Adjusting your Document Holder

The term document holder refers to the device that holds up documents you refer to as you sit at your desk and type. Many people don't have a document holder. They simply put reference material on the desktop. When they need to refer to it, they lean over.

If you frequently look down and to the side to review documents and reading material, you may well benefit from a document holder. Seeing the reference documents at eye level keeps your head and neck more neutral and centered. I recommend an adjustable 18-inch document holder (3M makes a great one) to position between your keyboard and monitor.

Not everyone can fit a document holder underneath the monitor. If this is the case, position the document holder approximately the same height and distance as the monitor. This will assist with visual tracking and minimize the need to re-focus when scanning between the documents and the screen.

Adjusting Your Monitor

Aside from the sitting considerations mentioned in the previous chapter, I believe there are two other reasons why so many computer workers lean or perch forward so frequently. The first has to do with focal distance, and the second is with what I call "the work hard fallacy."

It's always better to adapt the environment to the person than the person to the environment.

Although most people don't consider focal distance when they sit down to work, they nevertheless position themselves at the optimal viewing distance for reading text on their computer monitors, usually by leaning in or perching forward on their chairs so their heads are closer to the monitors. What they should do is adjust the position of their monitor and chair first, instead of adjusting themselves to fit the monitor. Leaning and perching forward puts additional, unnecessary stress on your body.

It's always better to adapt the environment to the person than the person to the environment. That means scooting your chair as close to the desktop as possible while still being able to work comfortably with your keyboard and mouse, and then adjusting your focal distance, the distance between your eyes and your monitor.

With your chair set up appropriately, bring the monitor several inches closer while viewing text on the screen; then move your monitor further away. (Better yet, have someone else move the monitor while you sit in your typing position.) As you move the monitor closer and further away, notice the subtle movements in the muscles of your eyes, neck, and face. Keeping your head positioned over the pelvis, find the distance that gives you the most comfort, softness, and relaxation in these areas. It's important to take time with this inquiry, to find the right position and fit of the monitor, for once you do find it, you won't need to change it again, unless your visual acuity changes. As you age, your visual acuity decreases, making it necessary to readjust your focal point.

Options to help you see more clearly include adjusting the size of the letters on the screen, adjusting the font, and seeing an optician to find the right prescription of computer glasses for you. The majority of desktop monitors are 19 inches tall. Yet, the smaller the monitor, the closer it should be to your eyes; the larger the monitor, the further away it should be away.

When sitting upright and reading text on a monitor, your gaze will typically slope approximately 10 to 15 degrees from your eyes downward to the screen. Ideally, your eyes should land at the base of the upper third of the screen. When positioned properly, the top of your head is approximately the height of the top of the monitor.

The "Work Hard Fallacy"

There seems to be an unconscious belief among some people that more effort equals more efficiency. I call this the "work hard fallacy." Somewhere during our evolution and socialization, we learned to associate muscle effort with success and proficiency. The idea goes something like this: The harder you work at your job, the more approval, praise, and success will come your way.

Probably many people learned these ideas at a very young age from caregivers, teachers and peers who rewarded them with praise and approval for working hard. The more effort we applied in school, the more we felt like good boys and girls, especially when our efforts were well received.

The personified posture of the hard-working office worker is one of a person sitting at the edge of the seat, head rounded or protruding forward, eyes glued to the monitor screen, the breath inhibited, and the fingers typing hard and fast at the keyboard. In reality, the office worker who is sitting in a relaxed and composed posture with minimal tension in his or her body is likelier to be more efficient.

During our evolution and socialization, we learned to associate muscle effort with success and proficiency.

The worker who perches forward, tenses their jaw, and has their eyes glued to the monitor while typing with a great deal of force is by no means more efficient than the person who is sitting in a composed and comfortable posture in their chair, with their jaw, neck and head completely relaxed and their head positioned over their pelvis. This person's body is not as run down at day's end.

That means that more muscle effort equals less efficiency and productivity. When driving in traffic or running late, it is a matter of instinct to tense, contract, and overuse your muscles. Your mind gets tricked into thinking that time moves faster and that you are being more productive when you exert more effort. Tension and stress narrows attention, and narrowed attention makes time seem to go faster. This leads to the fallacy that more tension and stress equates to a higher state of productivity.

As humans spend more and more time in the office gazing at the computer screen, putting an end to the "hard work fallacy" is paramount. Humans need to develop an awareness of how they use their bodies to end the rampant rise of overuse injuries.

5

Balancing the Towards
vs. Away Personality

People tend to "lean towards" what they want both physically and energetically. And some people's energy and physical posture "leans away." In general, towards people are motivated by goals, rewards, and fulfilling unmet needs. They have "type A," competitive, outgoing, ambitious, impatient, and sometimes aggressive personalities. They may put more effort into the things they believe in. Away people want to avoid being in the way. They want to avoid unforeseen problems. An away person's physiology is to lean back or away from life, and this can cause him or her to slouch more in the chair.

Who Has a Towards
and Away Personality?

How can you tell who has a towards and who has an away personality? I believe there is a unique feeling signature we have with every person we interact with, and this feeling signature causes us to lean toward or lean away. These feelings may fluctuate depending upon who or what we are dealing with. Some interactions with people cause us to want to lean in closer to them; other interactions make us want to lean away.

Think about how it feels to stand next to your best friend. How is your posture — forward, away, or balanced? How about your boss? How about your mother? How about a stranger who passes you walking down the street? The way we feel inside is always situational. And the way we feel always has an effect upon our posture. Just the opposite is true as well where our postures (as well as the postures of those around us) has an effect upon the way we feel.

Notice how the posture of the people in your environment affects the way you feel inside. Does sitting with them make you feel more constricted inside or make you want to pull away? Or does it make you want to lean in closer? Oftentimes when people have constricted breathing in their chest and lungs, perhaps due to perfectionistic ideas or their desire to be a good worker, they tend to unconsciously, without rhyme or reason, match or mirror these traits. Who makes you feel more open and relaxed? How is their breathing, posture, and emotional availability?

There is no judgement on either posture, towards or away. But your physical (and mental) strength and power comes from a balanced, aligned posture centered between the two extreme of towards and away. This ideal posture is centered between the heads of your two sit bones.

Benefits of a Balanced Posture

Some of the benefits of a balanced posture include:

- Spine aligned and your weight distributed throughout muscles more evenly

- Optimal posture for volitional and intentional action

- Feelings of confidence and strength

If you tend to be a "towards" person, here are some suggestions. Practice softening and allowing.

By "allowing" I mean to let yourself surrender to the organic rise and flow of events around you. Let the words on the screen float out to meet your eyes inside of their sockets, rather then leaning forward or reaching with your eyes to meet the words.

Whether you're an "away" or a "towards," find a more balanced and aligned posture. The shift can be come about by adapting your

---

mind or from changing your posture! If you lean your posture in the direction of "away," take a more proactive stance. Whether your head is forward or towards the back of your pelvis when sitting or standing, begin to reposition yourself over your pelvis. A lumbar support can help with this, for the position of the lumbar spine is reciprocal to the position of the cervical spine. When one goes forward, the other goes back.

Making these shifts consciously from within is a good first step. However, the change will be long lasting only if you incorporate the changes into our subconscious. As you begin to make subtle shifts from within, notice the interactions around you change as you engage with strangers, co-workers, and peers. I understand it's easier said than done! Especially since your "away" or "towards" habit was likely instilled and subcorticalized over the course of many years.

Standing Exercise:

Finding Balance

This exercise will help you achieve balance when you stand.

1. While standing, notice how your weight is distributed on your feet. Is it more towards the front of your feet or more toward the heels?

2. Imagine someone placing their hands softly above your head and ever so gently pushing down through the crown of your head. How would your weight shift? What would happen in your torso? Would your torso move to the right or left? Forward or backwards? Where is your line of gravity where the weight travels from your head down to your toes? Notice as well whether your weight is heavier over the right foot or the left (or is the weight distributed evenly)? Notice if the weight is more on the outside edge of your feet or on the inside?

3. Rock your weight forward toward your toes, keeping your spine aligned and straight and your gaze soft.

4. Rock your weight back towards your heels. Go back and forth like this several times.

5. Stop in the middle.

6. Notice where your line of gravity is. Has the weight shifted slightly forwards on your feet?

7. Cross your right foot over your left. Rock your weight steadily forward and back four or five times.

8. Uncross your legs. Pause and notice the differences. How is the weight distribution now through your feet?

9. Cross your right foot over your left and rock your weight steadily right and left four or five times.

10. Uncross your legs and rest. Notice now how your

weight is distributed between your two feet? Where is your line of gravity? Notice if you're bearing more weight on one foot than the other. (Take a brief rest in sitting before going on to the next step.)

11. Stand-cross the left foot over the right. Shift your weight forward and back slowly four or five times. Pause. Then shift your weight right and left four or five times.

12. Uncross your legs. Sense and notice the differences, and then sit down and rest.

13. Stand up again just to observe the differences. Feel how much more balanced and steady you feel?

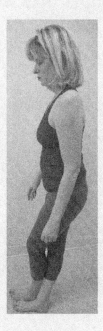 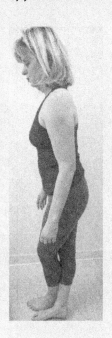

The Eyes

The eyes have it as far as working is concerned. Many people spend hours a day looking into their computer monitors. For that reason, making your workplace comfortable for your eyes is essential. This chapter looks into what you can do to make seeing — and seeing for long periods of time — easier and more comfortable.

Exploring Right-Eye, Right-Side Dominance

We live in a right-handed world. Approximately ninety percent of the world's population is right-handed. For this reason, most everyday items are designed for use by right-handed people. Manufacturers make scissors for left-handed people, but they don't make tools and household items for lefties. Even cars are designed mostly for right-handed usage in the United States. Most all keyboards are designed for right handedness, and the position of the mouse is most often on the right side of the keyboard.

Most people are also right-eye dominant. Follow these steps to find your eye dominance:

1. Hold your hands several inches in front of your face.

2. Make a triangle by touching your fingers and thumbs.

3. Look through this triangle.

4. Note the point that you see when you look through the center of the triangle.

5. Close your right eye and notice if the point moves. Then do the same with the left eye.

Whichever eye sees the point inside of the triangle is your dominant eye. It's worth noting, however, that not everyone has a dominant eye. Moreover, not everyone sees primarily through their dominant eye.

Discovering, and Breaking, Bad Work Habits

We need habits. Habits help us make our morning coffee, put on our socks and shoes, and drive ourselves to work safely and with ease. However, when inefficient habits become ingrained, we slowly lose the natural grace, flexibility, and ease of movement that our bodies and minds once knew. As we become "locked" in to our movement habits, the amount of movement options available to us decreases. Less movement options can lead to more rigidity, tightness, and lack of coordination.

Next time you start typing at your computer, notice some of your unconscious habits. For example, is your breathing inhibited? Do you tilt your head to the right as you type (as opposed to keeping your head in the middle)? Do you clench your jaw, raise your shoulders towards your ears, tighten your buttocks muscles, or furrow your brows? What other unhelpful habits do you notice?

With right eye dominance, most of us orient our heads and skeleton more to the right, expanding the awareness of our world around us on the right side. For this reason overuse injuries are much more common on the right side of the body. After you figure out your eye dominance, notice which way your eyes and head veer naturally. If you are right eye dominant, you might find the natural resting position of your eyes and head to be more to the right.

When your eyes look to the right, left, up, or down, your skeletal bones and structures follow accordingly. For many right-handers like me, due to my right hand and right eye dominance as well as society's encouragement of right-handedness, I overuse my right side. I do this habitually and excessively. As a result, I am more prone to overuse injuries on this side, and sometimes my shoulder feels sore.

I have come to believe that left-handed people have a slight advantage because they had to learn to survive in a right-handed world. They had to learn to some degree at least to be ambidextrous. You can find out how locked you are into habits of right handed usage by trying to perform tasks such as mousing, turning a key, or brushing your teeth on the left or non-dominant side of your body. How difficult performing these tasks is indicates the degree to which you are locked into your habits of right-handed usage.

A dominant-side body organization is perfectly normal and common. However, overtime, It can greatly affect the body's symmetry, balance, and overall function. Overusing certain muscle groups and under-utilizing others can eventually lead to discomfort and pain.

What Is Good Posture?

The definition of good posture according to Moshe Feldenkrais is the ability to organize yourself for action instantly and spontaneously in any direction and at any time. In other words, someone with good posture is ready to move out of the way when danger nears. Hence, some semblance of symmetry is important.

The key to achieving more symmetry is balance. That is one reason why positioning frequently-used items on both sides of our body is recommended.

If you use a document holder next to the monitor to view documents as you work, consider alternating sides for the holder. This way you look consistently to the left as much as you look to the right. If you are reaching to the right for the mouse all day, consider switching the mouse to the left side of your body. Consider as well placing other frequently used items on the left or less frequently used side throughout the day.

This same idea holds true for the neck and head. If you are a "hunt and peck typist" who looks down at the keys continually, be sure to counterbalance this by looking up to a similar percentage and degree. You can raise the monitor slightly to establish this balance.

The same idea also holds true for stretching. Stretch yourself in the opposite position of how you consistently hold yourself. If you slouch forward, frequently extend your neck, arms, and torso backwards. If you have a tendency to flex your wrists as you type, stretch your wrists into full extension. If you twist or turn your body to one side frequently, attempt to do the same action in the opposite direction.

During Feldenkrais lessons, a new pattern of organization takes place which can assist with this symmetrical realignment. As you listen to the lessons that accompany this book, first notice your habits. Then, with a childlike mindset, freely explore new alternatives of movement. Moving slowly and taking frequent rest breaks allows the nervous system to incorporate the change and reorganize itself accordingly.

Techniques for Relaxing the Eyes and Easing Headaches

Eyestrain is common to all computer workers. Staring at a computer screen for long periods of time is extremely tiring on the eyes. Long hours in front of the monitor may narrow your visual field and cause you to block out the world around you. It dampens your senses as well as your connection to the outside world. As your visual field narrows, so too may your overall awareness.

Long hours in front of the monitor may narrow your visual field and cause you to block out the world around you.

Tips for Easing Eyestrain

Here are some brief eye exercises you can do in the course of the day to relieve eyestrain:

- Rub your palms together quickly to create friction and heat, and then rest your palms over your eyes for several moments to allow your eyes to relax with the darkness and warmth. This is called "palming." Palming can be useful for easing the muscular tension around your eyes.

- Massage around the region of your temples and forehead to ease the tension and tightness that tends to cumulate in these regions.

- Refocus your eyes on an object twenty feet away every twenty minutes or so. This allows the muscles that are being overused (the near-sighted muscles) and the bands the holds the eyeball in the socket to relax.

- Blink frequently. Blinking provides additional lubrication to your eyes. (Computer users tend to blink less frequently when gazing for periods of time at a monitor screen.)

Eye Exercise:

Expanding Your Peripheral Vision

The following simple eye exercise can help to open and widen your visual peripheral field. As your peripheral field widens and softens, so too may the rest of your body. For this exercise, it's crucial that you move your eyes extremely slowly and smoothly, avoiding any jerky movements of the eye. If you get frustrated or tired, pause and take a rest at any time.

1. With eyes closed, very gently turn your head to the right, and then to the left, staying solely in your range of comfort and ease. Notice how far your head rotates in each direction. Notice as well if your head can rotate further in one direction. To which side does your head turn easier?

2. With your eyes still closed, notice in which direction your eyes naturally veer when you turn your head.

3. Keeping your eyes closed, imagine your eyes are a beach ball floating on the horizon of the ocean. While keeping your head still, float this beach ball to the upper-left corner of your visual field. Then smoothly float the ball down to the lower-left visual field. Continue this three movement times. If you are right-hand or right-eye dominant, chances are your movements are more jerky and you have a smaller range of motion on the left side.

4. If you notice any jerky or uneven eye movements, slow it down. See if you can iron out these jerky movements. Make your movements smooth and straight.

5. Float your eyes back and forth from the upper-left corner to the lower-left corner three times, then return the ball back to the center and take a brief rest. At this point it is interesting to retest the head rotation and see if it's easier to rotate your head to the left. If you find you are getting a headache from this exercise or your

headache is getting worse, you are likely exerting too much muscle effort. It simply means that you are likely having a difficult time breaking up the coordination patterns of the muscles around your eyes. Take a break from this exercise and try it again later. With practice, you will get it.

6.   Repeat Steps 3 through 5, but this time perform this exercise on the right side. Imagine floating the beach ball up to the upper-right quadrant of your visual field, then down to the lower-right visual quadrant. Perform this sequence three more times, going slowly. Perform the actions until the movement becomes as smooth as if you were spreading frosting on a cake.

7.   Take a rest and then float the beach ball (your eyes) clockwise into a full and complete square, through all four corners of your visual peripheral field — upper-right, lower-right, lower-left, and upper-left. Perform this action three times in the clockwise direction.

8.   Take a rest and then reverse the direction so your eyes move counter-clockwise. Do this three times. See if you can make the square even larger.

9.   Open your eyes and notice the shift in your peripheral vision. How much more open and expansive is it? How about the position of your shoulders? Notice if the rest of you feels more open and expansive as well.

Often times throughout my day, I perform this exercise solely to my left visual field, drawing a straight line from the center to the left five to ten times. Or I draw the line from the upper-left quadrant and then down to the lower-left quadrant several time. This exercise helps to increase my neck range of motion to the left and it increases my overall awareness and usage of my left side. This assists my overall balance and symmetry.

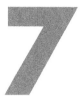

Posture

This chapter explores how the extensor and flexor postures evolved and how to tell when you are in the extensor or flexor posture. It explains why extensor and flexor responses can cause pain, what co-contracting muscles are, and how set points regulate the nervous system. Finally, this chapter offers a meditation exercise to help you let go of pain in your body.

The Flexors and the Extensors

When you feel sadness, worry, shame, anxiety or stress, the natural reaction is to contract your limbs and torso toward the center of your body. Let's call this the "flexor posture" because the action of your body in this state is akin to flexing your muscles. You tighten up. You contract as if you wanted your muscles to act as body armor.

When you feel alarm, fear, or a sudden urgency, the natural reaction is to extend your limbs and in effect pull away from our core. I call this the "extensor posture" because the action of the body in this state is to extend itself in the manner that some animals do when they want to look bigger. In the state of alarm and fear the natural reaction is to make yourself bigger and thereby make yourself look dangerous and more formidable to aggressors.

In the typical fight or flight reaction, an initial engagement of the extensors often occurs as you "freeze in your tracks" (like a deer in the headlights of an oncoming car). This is followed by the engagement of the flexor response as you flee as fast as you from the danger.

A Close Look at the Extensor and Flexor Postures

The extensor and flexor postures evolved because they were necessary for human survival:

- The extensor muscle reaction (a byproduct of alarm, fear, and urgency) evolved so that one would be ready and alert to danger. Our prehistoric ancestors had to be alert to predators and sudden changes in their environment. The extensor muscle reaction evolved to meet these challenges.

- The flexor muscle reaction (a byproduct of sadness, worry, shame, anxiety, and stress) evolved for self-protection. In the flexor posture, the mother hardens herself to protect the child in the womb and the warrior flexes his muscles to ward off blows from an enemy.

You can tell when you are in the extensor posture by observing these signs:

- You start to grow pale. Paleness occurs because the blood goes to your core, away from the superficial regions of the skin.

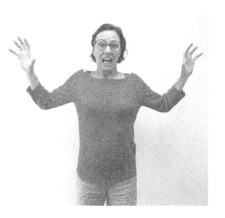

- Digestion slows or stops. Upper-intestinal action ceases in a state of fear and anxiety.

- The anal sphincter is pinched or constricted.

- The pupils dilate.

- Your peripheral vision widens and sharpens.

- The muscles on the back side of your body contract. These muscles are there to pull us backward, away from danger.

- Breathing becomes slowed and inhibited. Ribs become less mobile.

- Overworking of extra-ocular muscles (muscles around the eyes)

- Neck extensor muscles

- Flat thoracic spine

- Stiff and rigid chest wall-inhibited breath in this region

- Overworking of para-spinals of low back

- Tightness in gluteals

- Toes pointed outwards/heels pointed towards one another

- Toes hyper-extended

- Momentary halting of breath

  You can tell when you are in the flexor posture by observing these signs:

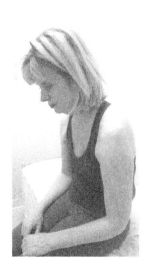

  - Increased heart rate with an accelerated pulse

  - Increase breathing rate

  - Heavy sweating with flushing as a result of the blood vessels dilating

  - A high metabolism

  - Tunnel vision (a loss of peripheral vision)

  - Neck rounded forward

  - Chest wall is pulled down towards the pubic bone-Breathing slowed and labored

  - Back rounded resulting in a slight winging of the inferior border of the scapula off the thorax

- Pelvic bone rounds more inwards

- Toes pointed inwards/heels pointed more outwards

- Toes curled under

- Paradoxical breathing with labored and shortened breaths

- Inhibited peristalsis

- Decreased lymphatic flow and circulation of fluids to one's organs as well as to the distal extremities.

Problems Caused by Engrained Extensor and Flexor Responses

When danger is imminent we reflexively employ these responses. These "fight or flight" response patterns that have been imperative to the survival of our species. However, the problem only occurs when we become so locked into these somatic responses, even when no enemy or danger is in sight.

For most of us, by the time we are our age, the musculoskeletal and physiological patterns of the extensor or flexor response are already so ingrained into our subconscious, we come to believe that this is simply who we are. We forget the freedom and ease of movement that we once knew as a child.

We become unaware that we walk with our gluteals held tight, our extensors of our back and neck over contracting, and our eyes and eye lids held vigilantly open. By the time patients come to see me with pain, these patterns are already so interwoven into the fabric of their persona as a result of years of programming from their former years.

Balancing the Extensors and Flexors

Good sitting, standing, walking, and lying down depend on the flexors and the extensors being in balance. Without this proper balance, certain muscles work at a shortened length; other muscles become overextended. Not only that, certain vertebra (which attach to the muscles) rotate too much and others rotate too little. This eventually results in an over utilization of some muscles and an underutilization of

---

others, an imbalance that can over time lead to body aches and pains.

If you've experienced longstanding chronic pain which has now become systemic, ask yourself if you are holding, bracing, and protecting yourself more than you need to.

Good sitting, standing, walking, and lying down depend on the flexors and the extensors being in balance.

Like all of us, people with chronic pain contract the muscles (for example) of their neck, back, and stomach to move, but when the movement is complete, they usually don't voluntarily relax the muscles. The muscles don't return to their full length. They don't return the muscles back to the state of rest.

People with chronic pain also tend to contract excessive musculature rather than solely engaging the muscles that are needed for the task at hand.

Co-contraction

Co-contraction occurs when a muscle needed for an action and its opposing muscle (the agonist and antagonist) contract simultaneously against one another. For example, co-contraction occurs when you contract the biceps and the triceps simultaneously when holding a glass of water in front of you. For a brief and short period of time, co-contraction is useful to stabilize your arm in this position.

The problem becomes when you contract both the flexors and extensors unnecessarily, as you often do when contracting both sides of a finger when mousing or typing, while holding it in the air over the key. In time, this will result in overuse and fatigue. Or when facing sudden fear or trauma our muscles will co-contract and "lock up."

For the most part, this behavior is done unconsciously, out of your awareness. Co-contraction occurs most often in the muscles in the back of the throat, neck, fingers, toes, eyes, and back.

With long term co-contraction patterns, eventually the muscles fatigue. The result is a throb, an ache, or even worse, the muscles constrict or impinge a nerve. Many people contract their muscles unconsciously even while they sleep. The fingers, toes, and jaw are common areas where this occurs.

Letting Go of Aching Muscles

After a Feldenkrais session, I have witnessed clients experience the release of their unconscious muscular-holding patterns. A parasympathetic response sets in where the muscles that were co-contracting or overworking begin to relax, neural impulses begins to slow and regulate, and one's blood pressure and pulse rate lowers. This often has a cascading effect upon the entire nervous system.

Sometimes the nervous stays in this calm tranquil state, while other times the pain symptoms are briefly re-evoked and spasms or shooting neural symptoms occur. Please note, no one needs to be afraid of this neural response after a Feldenkrais session, as usually the reaction calms within several minutes.

No one is really sure what causes the spasms or shooting neural symptoms after the "letting go" process. My theory is that the spasms are the body's attempt to keep "holding on." Out of habit, the body wants to maintain the familiar homeostatic state. The nervous system tends to cling to the known and steer away from the unknown. It strives to maintain a homeostatic set point for every physiological aspect of the body, including those habitual contraction and tension patterns.

How Set Points Regulate the Nervous System

Our neural set points began forming in our early years. Even before a person begins speaking, his or her fear and anxiety responses began to take shape. Whatever the circumstances — being left alone, mom and dad fighting, fears of the unknown — the blood pressure, heart rate, the contraction of the muscle fibers, the pressure on the diaphragm, the peristalsis of the colon, and all other neurological responses began to regulate accordingly.

As an infant, at the same time as you learn to model the behaviors and actions of your caregivers, you concurrently develop your own strategies for receiving love, acceptance, and belonging. You learned how to keep yourself safe in times of perceived danger and how to stay out of harm's way. These response patterns from your youngest years lay the foundation for how you use your body today. They lay the groundwork for the development of your neural set points.

The nervous system has a good reason for "holding on" to these old familiar set points. After all, when you were a young child in times of stress, these reactive somatic responses served an important purpose. They protected you from harm and gave you reassurance that you would make it through. These set points you developed became the stable "knowns" in a world of the "unknowns."

Your pre-programmed set points determine how closely your bones articulate with one another, the degree to which you sag your shoulders and neck, and the degree to which you hold your legs closer to one another while walking, standing, and sitting.

The good news is that the nervous system's set points can be re-regulated at any point in your life. All it requires is the will to change and a few helpful tools. You can teach the nervous system an alternative way of being — a new framework and foundation for

Reversing Body Patterns of Pain and Anxiety

In order to reverse the body patterns of pain and anxiety, you must at a subcortical level do the following:

- Learn the proper role of the flexors and extensors.

- Learn how to reduce unconscious and unnecessary habits of co-contraction as well as excessive effort in accessory muscles groups.

- Learn how to engage more of the core muscles to help take the load off of the distal muscles.

- Learn how to relax even the finest twitch-muscles of your eyes, toes, pinkies, gluteal (buttocks) muscles, and adductor (hip) muscles, as well as the muscles that put undue pressure on your internal organs (if they are contracting unnecessarily).

Journaling Exercise:

Letting Go of the Pain

Before you begin to "let go," it's important to remind yourself precisely what it is that you're holding onto. Only then can you take the triumphant first step forward in the direction of change.

1. Get in touch with what your pain is costing you. To do that, create as clear a picture as possible of the pain and how it's affecting your life. What is it costing you?

    •   Quality time with your children
    •   The ability to exercise, go for long walks, and ice skate
    •   Tolerance of your spouse's lack of assertiveness
    •   Ability to work longer hours
    •   The ability to focus
    •   Difficulty sleeping through the night

2. Ask yourself what you need to renounce or let go of in order to release the pain. Following are some suggested answers to this question. At first your answer may be very logical and linear, but try to determine what might be hiding underneath your answer. To help you determine what is hiding, you can ask "What else?" after each answer. Make a list of your answers. In Step 4 you will let go of the items on your list.

    •   "My need to be right." What else?
    •   "My need to control." What else?
    •   "My fear of what people think of me." What else?
    •   "My stress around finances." What else?

3. Visualize what your life might be like if you were free of the pain. Create as clear a picture as possible. See it in present time. You answers might include:

    •   I can sleep through the night.
    •   I see myself standing more confidently and solidly on my two feet.

- I have what feels like more time in the day.
- I feel more spaciousness inside of me.
- I feel a mildly cool breeze on my face on a nice summer day.
- I feel peace and joy inside.

As you state or write each one, pause and take a moment to envision it. See it. Feel it. Breathe it in.

4. Visualize yourself letting go each item you listed in Step 2. Release each item on your list one by one. Take time with this. And if anything else crosses your mind that you wish to release, go ahead and release that as well.

   - See yourself holding a helium balloon representing the first item on your list. See yourself letting go of the balloon and letting it rise up and away from you. When it floats up towards the sky, imagine it popping into a million pieces to be recycled back into the universe, and away and off of you. Do this for each item on your list.

5. Visualize all the remaining pain in your body, gather it all up, and then, rising like a helium balloon, let it slowly gravitate out of your physical body, up and away, out of the solar system and as far away from you as possible. If you prefer, you can visualize it popping into a million pieces after it leaves your body and enters the outer hemispheres.

6. Breath into how light, liberated, and free your body now feels.

Close your eyes and create a vision of how you can take this peaceful inner state with you as you continue on throughout your day.

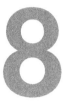

Sleep

E verybody craves a good night's sleep. Sleep is necessary for mental as well as physical good health. This chapter looks at the role sleep plays in healing and offers advice for getting a good night's sleep. You'll find an exercise to help you get to sleep, instructions for choosing a mattress and pillow, and advice specific for side sleepers, back sleepers, and stomach sleepers.

Sleep and Its Role in Healing

Throughout the night, your body cycles through stages of REM (rapid eye movement) and non-REM sleep. A typical sleeper experiences three 5-to-15 minute states of non-REM sleep followed by REM sleep. REM sleep is the phase where dreams occur.

During the third or last stage of non-REM sleep, delta waves of relaxation calm the sleeper's brain wave activity. In this stage, the body is able to

- Repair and regenerate soft tissue structures
- Build bones, tendons, and ligaments
- Strengthen the immune system

The third or last stage of non-REM sleep is the most crucial one for restoration and healing. It lasts about 20 to 30 minutes. It is sometimes called "slow wave" sleep because brain activity slows down during this stage.

Significant increases in the levels of beta-endorphin, norepinephrine, and dopamine occur. These hormones are linked to feelings of expanded mental clarity, happiness, and optimism. Growth hormones are also released in the third or last stage of non-REM sleep. Even if your lifestyle doesn't permit you the luxury of a full eight hours of sleep, a few hours of delta waves or restorative sleep will trick your brain into thinking it's had all the sleep it needs.

> The third or last stage of non-REM sleep is the most crucial one for restoration and healing.

Ironically, many sleeping pills deprive the individual of restorative non-REM sleep. In the long run this can heighten the experience of pain the next day. When our quality of sleep is low, even our perception of pain increases.

Sleep and the Pain Cycle

Unfortunately, when people enter the "pain cycle," disturbances in slow, restorative sleep usually result. And if they carry stress, fears, and anxieties from the day into the subconscious world of their sleep, restorative sleep is even less likely.

A lack of restorative sleep reinforces states of muscle tension and stress, further preventing the body from truly relaxing. After a few days of non-restorative sleep, the deprived sleeper experience's a lack of focus and mental clarity and over time may experience generalized muscle pain.

> A lack of restorative sleep reinforces states of muscle tension and stress

Tips For Getting A Good Night's Sleep

Here are some tips for getting a good night's sleep:

- Develop a routine of transitioning from your busy work day and life into a state of peaceful calm from the moment you enter your bedroom.

- Before going to sleep, avoid anything that causes stress or fear. For example, avoid horror and action films or laborious computer work.

- Make your bedroom into a sanctuary of safety, tranquility, and restfulness.

- Avoid bright colors and strong lighting in your room. Choose soft color tones for you place of sleep. Replace neon light bulbs with soft incandescent or color-adjustable LED light bulbs.

- Play calm music as opposed to upbeat tunes prior to sleep.

- If that chatter of your "monkey mind" won't stop and prevents you from falling asleep, first acknowledge your thoughts rather than ignore them and pretend that they just don't exist. Tell your mind that you hear its thoughts, worries, and fears, and you will address them tomorrow or another time. Just not now. Silence your mind. Imagine turning the dial to your thoughts off, as if turning down a dial or flipping off a light switch.

- Think positive thoughts prior to sleep. Think of three things positive things that happened to you during the day and the role you played in them. When we go to sleep with positive thoughts and feeling, they will gradually permeate into the land of our dreams. Our dreams are the period where neural connections and bonds are reformed and strengthened. Reinforcing positive thoughts and emotions into our subconscious sleeping states will set the stage for a more positive start of the next day.

Choosing a Pillow and Mattress

People often ask me to recommend a type of pillow or mattress. I recommend ones that are on the firmer spectrum and are organic, untreated, and non-synthetic. Mattresses made with synthetic ingredients release gas and chemicals into the air. Most mattresses contain polyurethane foam, Styrofoam, and polyester and are treated with fire retardants and chemicals that are recognized carcinogens. (There are no standard listings of chemicals on products, so it's important to check with the manufacturer or store prior to purchasing a pillow or mattress. Or shop at a natural and organic bedding store.) A critical part of staying in good health is choosing products for your home that are toxin-free.

Many people with sleep apnea, breathing difficulties, or heart problems prefer to sleep with two pillows or with their head higher up. They claim this position is more comfortable and easier to breathe. If this is true for you and sleeping in this position will help you to have a better night's sleep, then stick with it. Yet after

Sleep Exercise:

Ease Yourself Into A Good Night's Sleep

1. Lie on your bed or on the floor.

2. Make sure that the pillow or towel under your head is no more than one inch thick. The idea is to make sure your back and neck are straight and parallel to your bed or the floor.

3. Bend your knees, or if it makes you more comfortable, place a pillow under your knees so your knees are bent.

4. Think of a word (or phrase) that describes the essence or quality of that you as a person would like to emanate into the world. For example, your word could be wisdom, freedom, acceptance, love, abundance, health, vitality, fulfillment, generosity, happiness, or stamina.

5. Inhale, and as you do so, breathe in your word and all it represents for you.

6. On a long and slow exhale, release anything that is in the way of you embodying the essential quality your word describes. Draw this quality into the center of your heart.

7. Continue inhaling and exhaling, and with each exhale, release all that stands in the way of you embodying your word.

8. Sort of like a mantra, breathe in this quality as you expand your breath, and exhale anything getting in the way of you having this as you release this expansion.

9. You can add pelvic tilts, where you gently push through the soles of your feet and rock your tailbone up on the in breath, release and allow your back to gently arch on the out breath. This undulation motion will help to relax your nervous system.

performing some of the Feldenkrais lessons in this book, or the towel under the neck exercise, perhaps you can gradually retrain yourself to sleep with your head lowered and your spine in a more neutral alignment.

The biggest mistake most people make when they sleep is choosing the wrong pillow. A pillow that is too big or too small puts your head into a non-neutral posture. To decide the size of your pillow, first figure out the position that you sleep in a majority of the night, or at least the position you start off the night in. Because some people's cervical spine (or neck) protrudes forward of their spine more than others, the only way to find the correct size of the pillow is to try it out.

Posture for Sleeping

Finding the right posture for sleep is essential for avoiding pain and healing the body, especially the spine and neck. You spend about one third of your life in your bed. The rest of this chapter offers advice for finding the right sleeping posture.

Of course everyone tosses and turns throughout the night, so whatever position you start in, you may very well find yourself in another position when morning comes. That's understandable. Still, whatever position you hold your bones, ligaments, and skeleton in the longest leaves a strong imprint as to where you are training them to be.

Back Sleeper

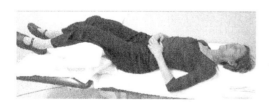

Back sleepers need a very thin or small pillow. Sometimes a towel's thickness is all you need. While lying on your back, if your head flexes forward or if your chin tilts even slightly downwards, your pillow is too high and needs to be lowered.

When sleeping on your back, place two pillows under your knees. This will support your lower back and make sure your low back is in a more flattened and relaxed state as you sleep. If you have back pain, putting a pillow under your knees is crucial. Even if you don't have back pain, I recommend sleeping with a pillow under your knees. It's a good practice to train yourself good postural habits before the pain or discomfort sets in.

Side Sleeper

Side sleepers need a thick pillow or a thin pillow doubled over. If your upper ear is closer to your upper shoulder than it is on the other side, your pillow is too thick. If you find your lower ear closer to your shoulder on the side you're lying on, your pillow is too thin and you need a thicker pillow. Adjust the pillow height so that your head is

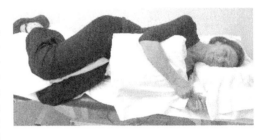

in a straight line from head to tail and your right shoulder is the same distance from your right ear as your left shoulder is from your left ear.

Another important tip for side sleepers: Place one pillow between your arms and one pillow between your knees. Or you can use a body pillow, which is a long pillow that fits between your arms and legs. Using pillows this way keeps your spine and pelvis in a more neutral alignment.

Stomach Sleeper

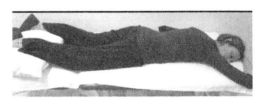

If you sleep on your stomach, a small or thin pillow is recommended. Or you may not need a pillow at all. This is how babies often sleep, and their spine remains neutral in this position. As we age and we begin to develop neck stiffness and limited range of motion this position becomes uncomfortable for many of us because of the pressures it places upon our neck.

Sitting in a Car

I know this chapter is called "Sleep," and I certainly wouldn't want you to fall asleep in your car. But I include this brief discussion of sitting in a car because many of us spend long periods of time in our cars commuting, and doing so, we develop back pain. The remainder of this chapter offers some pointers for preventing the pain from coming on.

Many people sit in the car with their chair positioned too far away from the steering wheel. As a result, especially if they drive with their hands at the top of the steering wheel, they drive with their elbows locked and sometimes their shoulders locked as well.

Rather than drive in this position, scoot your chair close enough to the steering wheel so your elbows are bent and rest towards the front of your torso. Your hands should be at the four o'clock and eight o'clock position on the steering wheel. Your grasp of the wheel should be firm yet soft.

If you have pain or neural symptoms throughout your arm, be sure to purchase an anti-vibratory steering wheel cover.

Another big mistake people make when they drive is to recline their chairs backwards. This inhibits the accessibility of the back, scapula, and pelvic regions, all of which are needed to turn the steering wheel and change gears (if your car is a stick shift model). Because of the forward and downward gravitational pull of the head and neck, the lower back and neck musculature have to work harder to keep the head and arms upright.

As the car shakes and vibrates, all the pounds of pressure go into the lower back (specifically, the area of the lower back that is most rounded backwards), when this pressure would otherwise be distributed throughout the spine. The discs between each vertebra act as shock absorbers, just as the shocks on your car do. The discs aid in the absorption of the vibratory forces, dampening them before they travel through the rest of the system. When the spine is rounded, however, these fluid-filled discs are pushed towards the back of the spine, decreasing their effectiveness as shock absorbers.

The best way to protect the spine and use your muscles in a bio-mechanically optimal way is to have your spine straight (in its natural S-shaped curve). Most cars are made with adjustable lumbar supports for keeping the spine straight.

If you have lower back pain or if the bone structure of your skeleton is quite rounded, you'll probably find this erect posture of your chair quite uncomfortable. Hence, I recommend you incrementally, little by little, bring your chair into a more upright position and incrementally increase the lumbar support. If your chair is reclined, no lumbar support is needed. Lumbar supports are really only helpful when the chair is almost upright or fully upright.

If you have lower back pain, any attempts to sit straighter will be uncomfortable if you maintain the same position for more than 30 minutes. Every 20 to 40 minutes, depending upon how bad the pain is, get out of your car and stretch.

Diet

A ny pain state held in the body for a prolonged period of time will result in nutritional deficiencies. You need nutrients to nourish and repair all parts of your body, including damaged nerves, damaged connective tissues, and sore muscles. Having to heal the body can increase your nutritional needs because so much effort has to go into healing.

Any pain state held in the body for a prolonged period of time will result in nutritional deficiencies.

Diet is an essential part of any wellness program. A healthy diet is a pertinent part of a healthy lifestyle for it will help you to feel more energized, happy, and alive. This chapter looks at how toxins get lodged in the body and the role of free radicals in inflammation. It shares some ideas about how to improve your diet so you can get on the road to good health.

Toxins in the Body

The body is equipped with its own self-regulating detoxification mechanisms. These mechanisms are designed to eliminate waste products, but they can only do so much. When your body is overloaded with excessive levels of toxins brought about by stress or other causes, your internal waste management system becomes overwhelmed, and this in turn can lead to a further increase in toxins.

The best way to prevent your body from being flooded with toxins is to discover why the toxins are accumulating in the first place. Something may have interfered with your body's ability to remove toxins. Culprits can include heavy metals and chemicals, food sensitivities, and immune challenges to the immune system from viruses, bacteria, or fungi, and other such issues as well.

A thorough nutritional exam can determine if toxins are accumulating in your body due to an impaired digestive tract or an attack from outside invaders such as Candida, parasites or environmental toxins. Determining an individual's food and supplement deficiencies and requirements can require many tests and procedures. Remember: your body is an integrated system. All the parts need to be in healthy communication with each other. In an integrated system it can be difficult to determine what causes an influx of toxins.

Any "itis" — for example, arthritis, colitis, and tendonitis — that has to do with inflammation is a sign of an overload of foreign substances in the blood. Besides the aforementioned diseases, carpal tunnel syndrome and irritable bowel syndrome can be caused by an accumulation of foreign substances. An anti-inflammatory diet is key to preventing these diseases.

Antioxidants for Combating Free Radicals

Fortunately, there are crucial changes you can make today, starting first and foremost with your diet. Strive for an anti-inflammatory, free radical-reducing diet that is right for you.

Free radicals are destructive byproducts of the body's own inflammatory response. Stress, environmental toxins, x-ray radiation, and immune activation can cause an increase in the production of free radicals. When free radical levels rise too high, the cells becomes overrun with inflammation, and this can lead to chronic medical problems. Free radicals destroy the cells' mitochondria, the cells' source of power, causing the cells to weaken and malfunction, resulting in an inflammatory response. This is why many anti-aging products aim to decrease free radicals in your body.

Antioxidants neutralize free radicals. Antioxidants are found in rainbow-colored foods such as carrots, berries, cantaloupe, and red and yellow peppers. They are also found in red kidney and pinto beans, garlic, artichokes, broccoli, kale, and dark leafy green vegetables. Vitamin C, vitamin E, beta-carotene (a precursor to vitamin A), some B vitamins, selenium, and green teas are all effective anti-oxidants.

Foods to Avoid

Foods that are high in hydrogenated or trans-fat increase free radical production and the body's inflammatory response. These foods include margarine, packaged foods such as cake mixes, fast foods, fried foods, doughnuts, pastries and snack foods. Any food that contains refined sugar and high-fat meats — in fact, any highly processed food — increases free radical production. Not only that, but foods that contain white sugar (that includes most refined foods) been stripped of their nutrients. This is why I recommend eliminating sugar, white flour, and processed food from your diet.

You should also avoid foods that contain high amounts of LDL, the so-called bad cholesterol. These foods include whole milk, cream, pastries, cheese (other than cottage cheese), and fried foods. Choose lean and healthy meats such as fish and chicken.

Strategies for Eating Healthily

If you are working with a buddy or have a partner you reside with, share with them your nutrition goals so they can help keep you accountable. Tell them one sugary, fatty, or processed food you wish to eliminate.

If you have a diet high in these sort of foods, make it your goal to eliminate one or more "bad" food item per week, or simply allow yourself to eat such foods only one time per week while eliminating them for the rest of the week.

Food has a strong emotional component. You may notice yourself reaching for certain foods when you are feeling certain emotions. For example, you may reach for carbs to calm your feelings of insecurity or rejection. Sometimes when you're feeling "high" on life with an excess of sensation you overeat to bring yourself back down to your baselines. Sometimes you eat faster or over eat to cover up certain feelings or emotions.

The goal is to eat healthily and consciously. Most people know what constitutes a healthy diet, yet in our stressed and busy lives we resort to quick and fast options. Grocery stores are filled with processed and unnatural foods that contain sugar, fat additives, preservatives, and other unhealthy chemicals. These foods impound your immune system and other internal processes.

Get in the habit of reading food ingredient labels. Be conscious of the foods you choose to eat, as well as the food while you are eating it.

Slow down and really chew your food. This will help with your digestion and allow your body to draw more nourishment from the food you eat.

Making healthy food choices every day is a way to empowerment. Choice is the key word here. Choose to make the outcomes of a healthy diet more important than the pleasure of simply eating food.

10

Foam Roller Exercises

The exercises in this chapter are great for anyone with mild back, hip, shoulder, or arm pain. They're great for anyone who works at a desk job. For that matter, they're great for anyone seeking more symmetry and comfort in his or her body. These exercises will help massage out the sore muscles of the back as well as help with the glide and movement of the scapula. They also help integrate the use of your arms with the rest of you.

White rollers are recommended. Blue, black or colored foam rollers are quite firm and are not recommended when starting out. If you are in pain I highly recommend using one or two thick towels rolled up into the shape of the spine as opposed to the 6 by 36-inch polyethylene foam rollers.

You want to remain comfortable throughout the duration of the exercises. Make sure your head is fully supported. If you're lying on towels, your pelvis will be on the ground; if you're using a foam roller, your pelvis should rest at the base of the roller.

When performing the exercises, avoid inhibiting your breath. Perform each exercise 5 to 7 times in a slow and steady manner.

Back-Lying Foam Roller Exercises

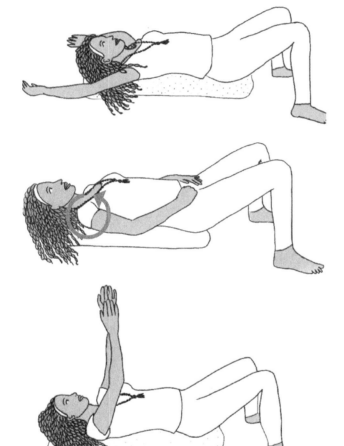

Snow Angels

Shoulder Circles

Arm Lengthening
Gently elongate one arm up towards the ceiling; then relax it back down to meet the other. Feel how your shoulder blade slides away from your spine with each elongation of your arm. Fingers remain soft and slightly curled. Palms stay in contact with one another at all times.

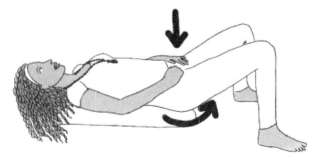

Pelvic tilts
Gently push through your feet in order to roll your pelvis up (your back will flatten). As you release, your back will arch. Inhale as you roll your pelvis up; exhale on the release. Perform this exercise in a rhythmic and relaxed manner as if you could perform it for an hour without getting tired.

Log Roll Side To Side
Roll your entire back left
and right to massage out
your back

(Optionally, you could
add a pelvic tilt as you
roll to each side)

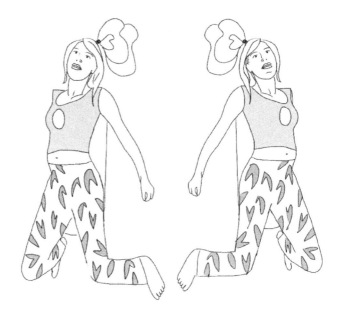

Roll off the foam roller and
lie on your back and rest.

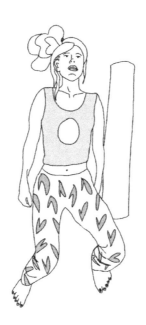

Side-Lying Foam Roller Exercises

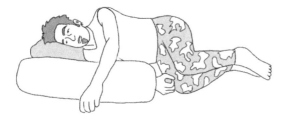

1. Lie on your right side with a pillow under your head, your knees bent 80 to 90 degrees and your wrist resting on the foam roller.

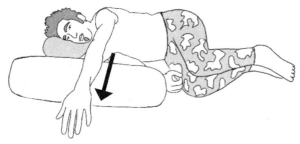

2. Gently initiating the movement from the shoulder blade region of your upper arm, roll the foam roller away from you, lengthening your arm. Perform this movement 5 times. Then rest.

You are mobilizing your scapula, freeing it up so it's more accessible for movement. Notice if your head and neck moved while you performed this exercise.

3. Perform the same movement five times without moving your head or neck. Rest.

4. Perform it 5 times with moving your head and neck; then rest.

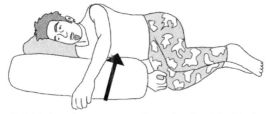

5. Gently initiating the movement from the shoulder blade region of your left arm, roll the foam backwards, towards your body as your upper shoulder gently rolls backwards. Perform this movement 5 times.

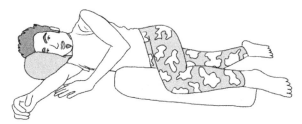

6. Move the foam roller down and place your upper knee and ankle onto it (you'll most likely need to straighten the bottom leg to move it out of the way).

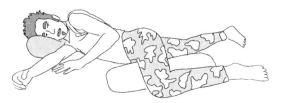

7. With your left leg, gently and effortlessly roll the roller forward away from your body, and then back towards your body. Notice if your torso and upper body moves along with you as you perform this movement. Pause

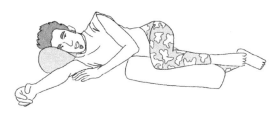

8. Then roll your leg backwards 5 times. Notice what your head and neck is doing. Rest for a few moments.

9. Then place the roller under both your arm and your leg. Roll your arms and legs forwards and backwards. Allow your head/neck to move along with the movement of the rest of you. Pause.

10. Continue the same movement 5 times yet this time inhibit the movement of your head/neck. Notice how it's more difficult to roll as far. Pause

11. Repeat step #9. And notice if it's easier to roll, and if more parts of you are now involved.

12. Lay on your back and rest. Feel how your body is now making contact with the floor. What's different? What part of your body is most in contact with the floor? What part is the least in contact?

13. Roll your head gently right, and then left. Feel which side it rolls to easier.

Roll to the other side and perform this same exercise on the other side of your body.

11

Nerve Stretching

I f you are feeling tingling, burning, numbness (known as parasthesias), especially in addition to muscle weakness, chances are you have some nerve involvement.   Nerves can get injured just like muscles, tendons, and ligaments.   Especially when there's scar tissue, inflammation, or a lack of blood flow to the region, nerves can get "trapped."

The key to get them moving again is to stretch them.   There are two main ways to stretch the nerve which I'll advise:

1.   One is known as the flossing technique where you rhythmically oscillate your hand & head back and forth into and out of the stretch for 3-5 repetitions.

2.   And the other is where you hold the stretch for 4-10 seconds three times.

The most important thing to know about doing the nerve stretching is you want to stop before you get to the point of discomfort. All you want to feel is a slight stretch, such as the sensation you feel in your hamstrings as you bend forward to touch your toes. Anything past that point will be too much and you could flair up your nerve for days.

For all the stretches start at level 1 and progress to the next level only if you can perform the full range of movement free of discomfort or irritation.

There are three main nerves in the arm. The Median, Ulnar and Radial.

Median Nerve Stretches

If you are experiencing parasthesias in this region of your hand:

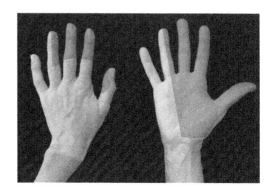

I recommend the following stretching protocol:

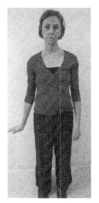
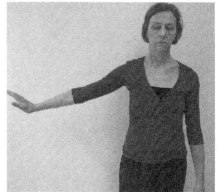

Level 1   Level 2

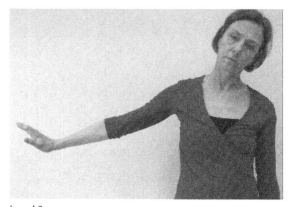

Level 3

Ulnar Nerve Stretches

If you are experiencing parasthesias in this region of your hand:

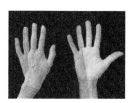

I recommend the following stretching protocol:

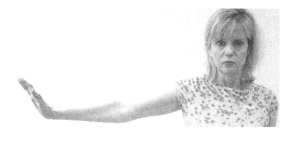

Level 2

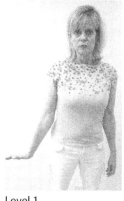

Level 1

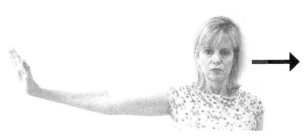

Level 3

First perform this stretch with your head in neutral, and if you are without an increase in any neural symptoms, side bend your head.

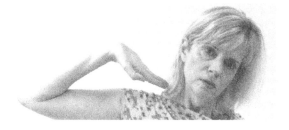

Level 4

First perform this stretch with your head in neutral, and if you are without an increase in neural symptoms, side bend your head away from your bent arm.

Radial Nerve Stretches

If you are experiencing parasthesias in this region of your hand:

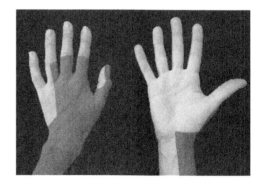

I recommend the following stretching protocol:

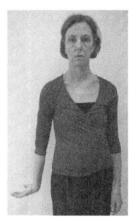

Level 1

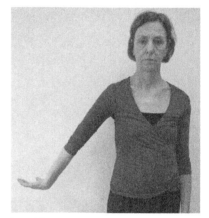

Level 2

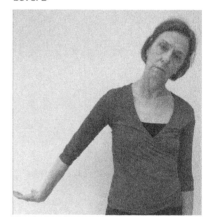

Level 3

After performing a series of the nerve stretching there may be a transient response of paresthesias or discomfort that should quickly resolve within a few minutes. If such symptoms last longer than this period of time, that means you've either stretched the nerve too far, or performed too many repetitions. If attempting such stretches again, go down one level, perform fewer repetitions, and/or hold the stretch for a shorter period of time.

These stretches could result in symptom relief and improved ease of movement when performed correctly.

12

Exercises for Relaxing the Neck and Jaw

The neck and jaw are two of the primary places where the body holds tension. This chapter presents some exercises to help you relax your neck and jaw.

Sometimes releasing the muscles around our jaw unravels and releases many other parts of the body. If you are in a lot of pain, doing stretches or other exercises in this book may be too painful. Hence, I recommend just starting with these simple jaw exercises.

Exercise To Ease Neck Aches And Pains

1. Lie on the floor on your back on a rug or a yoga mat with your knees bent, feet about hips width apart. Begin by gently rolling your head to the right and left to assess how far you can easily roll your head to each side.

2. Place a rolled-up small-to-medium sized towel in the nook of your neck. You can also use a roll of paper towels (approximately half to three-fourths of the roll) or even a balled-up item of clothing.

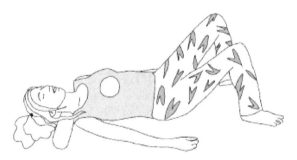

3. Perform a gentle and effortless pelvic tilt. Perform this rhythmic undulation several times. Make the movement so easy, so effortless, you could do it for an hour without getting tired. Perform about 15 repetitions and then pause and take a rest.

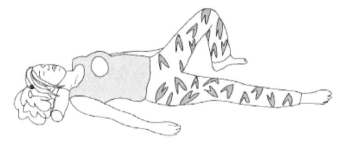

4. Roll halfway onto your side. Roll onto the side that is bothering you unless it's too painful to actually lie on this side. Roll the towel so it is a half roll thicker and place it under your neck.

5. Bend the opposite knee and place this foot comfortably on the ground. Lengthen the leg on the side you're lying on. Gently push through the standing foot in order to perform a gentle one-sided pelvic tilt. What that means is that you

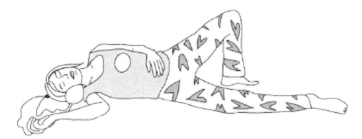

slightly unweight your pelvis from the ground as you roll it in the upwards direction. As you do this, you should feel the pressure on the towel roll slightly increase. Repeat this several times. Reposition the towel roll so it is directly on the area of discomfort.

6. Perform this rhythmic undulation about 15 times. Coordinate each pelvic tilt with your breathe. Inhale roll up; exhale release.

7. Pause. Remove the towel roll. Take a rest on your back and notice the differences.

8. Roll all the way onto your side, position your legs and the towel the same way with the knee of your standing foot pointing up in the direction of the ceiling, and perform the pelvic tilt series. Remember to give a gentle push through the standing foot, so the trajectory of the movement passes through the sole of the foot, then knee, then through your pelvis and torso, all the way through to the top of your neck and head. Using minimal muscle effort. The belly and chest should be completely free and relaxed. Gently undulating or mobilizing the head and neck gently in the upwards direction with each tilt of the pelvis.

9. Lay on your back, remove the towel roll, and rest with either your legs long or bent.

**If you are have headaches or upper neck pain, lie on your back and place the towel roll or a small rubber ball (such as a racquetball) at the base of your occiput (the place where your skull meets your neck) and perform several repetitions of the pelvic tilt from this position.

**If you are have a knot of tightness in your neck, shoulder or back place a scrunched up washcloth or a small rubber ball under this region. Reposition your body so the cloth or ball lies directly underneath. Then go ahead and perform one or two legged pelvic tilts. This will help to massage out this region of tension.

Exercise to Relax the Jaw & Neck #1: The Cork

You need a cork from a wine bottle or similar object such as a rolled up paper towel to do this exercise.

1. Place the cork in your mouth so you have a solid hold of it between your two lips. This will feel quite awkward at first, especially if you are one to hold your jaw/mouth tight.

2. Try swallowing once or twice.

3. See if you can maintain the cork in your mouth for 30 seconds to one minute.

4. Take out the cork and rest. You might notice instantly how your lips fall apart from one another and allow for a gap in the space of your mouth.

5. Place the cork back into your mouth. Imagine that the end of the cork which is pointed away from you is the tip of a pencil. Draw a line with this pencil straight up the wall, and then back down. Perform this 5 times in each direction. Make the line as straight as possible. Perform this movement without moving your head and neck.

6. Rest for a minute and then place the cork back into your mouth. With the imaginary tip of the pencil, draw a line straight right and then left (with the cork). Perform this five times in each direction.

7. Rest a minute. Then, keeping your head stationary, perform the same movement with the cork as you did in Step 6, but include the movement of the eyes. Move the end of the cork and your eyes synchronistically to the right, and then to the left. Perform this five times in each direction.

8. Rest. This time allow your head to roll with your eyes and jaw. Move the end of the cork and your eyes synchronistically to the right, and then to the left, allowing your head to roll along with this motion. Perform this five times in each direction.

9. Remove the cork and rest.

10. Place the cork back into your mouth, next lets coordinate the movement of the cork and eyes moving up and then down, yet keeping the head still. Perform this movement of the eyes and cork moving synchronously and smoothly up and then down, 5 times in each direction. Rest.

    *** As extra credit, if you get to the point of performing this step with ease, you could try taking the eyes and cork in opposite directions, making sure each movement is rhythmic and coordinated. As the eyes go up, the tip of the cork points down. And visa versa. Five times smoothly and coordinated.

11. Return to the movement of gliding the eyes and the tip of the cork smoothly up and down, yet this time include the movement of the head and neck. That means gently move the jaw, eyes, and head up and down synchronously and slowly, 5 times in each direction.

Notice what changes you experience around your jaw, neck, and face region as a result of performing these exercises.

***As a suggestion if you have TMJ or a habit of jaw tension, try keeping the cork in your mouth for a minimum of one minute while performing any daily task, such as washing the dishes, making the bed, or cutting vegetables.

Exercise to Relax the Jaw & Neck #2: Painting the Teeth

1. Lie or sit comfortably. Close your eyes. Notice which way your eyes are veering. Notice which way your nose and chin are veering.

2. Gently roll your head once to the left and once to the right, staying in the range of comfort and ease. Notice how easily it rotates to each side and which side it rotates to easier?

3. Imagine your tongue is a paint brush. Using your imagination, we are going to paint the left side of our teeth, starting on the inside upper row. What color would you like to paint your teeth?

4. Imagine dipping your tongue into the color paint you chose and then taking the tip of your tongue to the inside of the upper buck tooth just to the left of midline.

5. Paint that tooth up and down several times, taking note of the sensation that your tongue feels as it slides along the tooth. Notice the shape and texture of the tooth. Notice the ridges and unique nuances of this tooth. Rest.

6. Move one tooth to the left and paint the inside of the next tooth. Do this 3 to 5 times. Pause, and then move onto the next tooth on the left.

7. Moving one tooth at a time continue this exploration of painting, feeling, and noticing. Go slow. Repeat this until all the inside upper-left side of the teeth are painted.

Pause. Notice and appreciate any differences in how your mouth and face feels.

8. Now we're going to paint the outside of each tooth. Begin with the tooth closest to the midline and work, tooth by tooth, slowly out to the left. Feel free to take a rest at any time, especially if the movement becomes uncomfortable.

9. Repeat this until all the upper left teeth are painted. Rest. Take some time to really notice the changes that are happening inside of your mouth. How does the space between your teeth on the right side compare to that of the left?

10. Repeat steps 6 to 11 on the bottom left row of teeth. Take your time.

When you finish painting all of the teeth on the left side, compare the differences between both sides. Which side feels larger? Gently roll your head once to the right, and once to the left. Which way is it easier to roll?

Which way do your eyes veer now? How about your tongue? How about your nose? Notice the softness and openness on your left side of your cheek and face and compare how that feels different from the right. How about your shoulder blades and shoulders? Is there a difference between how your pelvis is making contact with the table or chair?

You can either leave this as a one sided lesson. One sided lessons can help you to better feel and clarify differences. Or, if you'd like, you can continue the same sequence on the other side.

13

Therapeutic Taping Techniques

Therapeutic Elastic taping (a cotton strip with an acrylic adhesive) has become a popular modality for treating a variety of physical disorders. Physical therapists, chiropractors, and athletic trainers use the tape. When applied properly, tape can help with the flow of blood and lymph, it can aid muscle facilitation and/or inhibition, and it may even alleviate pain and edema. A variety of brands are available over the counter, including rock tape, KX tape, Leukotape and kinesiology tape. The tape can also be used for stability and maintaining neutral postures.

This chapter presents two simple taping techniques I have found quite useful. You can apply these techniques on your own.

Encouraging the Wrist to Be in the Neutral Position

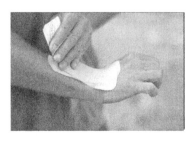

This first taping technique is great for anyone who experiences wrist pain and finds that they habitually use their wrists in non-neutral postures. Too much wrist flexion over time can result in "ligament laxity," or stretching of the ligaments on the back side of the wrist. When ligaments become stretched, finding neutral postures become much more difficult and bracing or taping techniques can then be helpful.

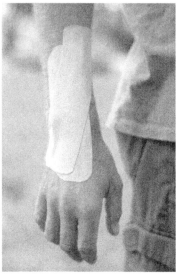

1. Cut two pieces of tape approximately 4 to 7 inches long.

2. Extending your wrist back beyond neutral (taking into account how the tape will stretch), tear the tape on one end and apply it to the mid back of the hand. Take off the adhesive as you apply it over the mid forearm.

3. Rub the tape back and forth to secure it. Heat helps the tape to stick. Two pieces are recommended to ensure the stability of this position.

With this usage, the brain is tricked into thinking that the tape is a part of the skin, and as the wrist is bent towards end range, the stretch reflex will be elicited signaling to the brain to stop the movement and to find neutral once again. The proprioceptive and kinesthetic properties of the tape provide relevant feedback to the brain as to where the wrist is in positioned in space and its relationship to the rest of the body both during movement and at rest. The tape will block the wrist from going into a shortened or lengthened position, which then allows the muscles and soft tissues time to rest and heal. Over time, the muscle memory for this more optimal position will be learned. Resting overworked and overstretched muscles and tendons is a first step towards recovery.

If you find you are bending your wrist too much ulnarly (or towards the pinky side), apply the tape over your dorsal radial (thumb side) of your wrist. Deviate your wrist radially, or in the direction of your thumb when applying.

Helping with Shoulder Pain

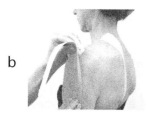

The second technique is helpful is for people with ligament weakness, subluxation, or pain around the shoulder. This technique helps support the head of the humerus into its socket, inhibits excessive muscle contraction (particularly around the upper trapezius), and helps with the normal glide of the scapula.

For this technique you'll need another person to help you with the application.

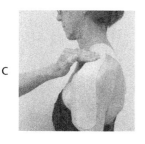

1. Cut three strips of tape approximately 6-7 inches long.

2. Anchor the first strip at the base of the shoulder blade. Gently remove the adhesive backing as you apply the tape in an upwards direction (along the medial border of the scapula) towards the region where the shoulder meets the neck, as demonstrated in photo a. After each piece is applied, rub the tape back and forth to secure it.

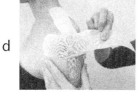

3. Apply the second strip at the lateral side of the arm, as shown in photo b. Provide upward tension or stretch on the tape until it passes over the shoulder joint. Release the tension for the remainder of the application.

4. Optionally, the client could sideband their neck away from the tape during application. This will help to lift the skin from the underlying fascia and decrease the work of the muscles.

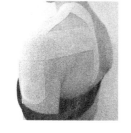

5. Optionally, apply a third strip anchoring it at the front of the shoulder joint. Secure it across the shoulder blade region as demonstrated in image e, until it meets the 1st piece of tape. (Be sure this piece doesn't cross to the other side of the spine).

For other taping techniques, please consult a professional. Some clients find it helpful to simply apply the tape over or around the parts of the legs or arms that are in pain. The tape is not to be used over open wounds. Avoid applying it so tight it constricts blood flow or limits movement.

a

b

c

d

e

14

Entering the Realm of the Pain Body

The natural tendency is to resist or pull away from sensations that don't feel good and to move closer to sensations that do feel good. We may try to distract ourselves from pain through work, addictions, keeping busy, or other avoidant behaviors. These distractions may work for a period of time, but in the end, the pain still remains. As the ole adage goes, "What you resist, persists." This is the absolute truth with pain. I have found that with pain (whether mental or physical) the only way to the other side is straight through.

This chapter presents a meditation to enter the realm of the pain body — free from judgement, shame, or resistance. The moment a story or judgement about the sensation enters, the neutrality of the sensation is drowned out. And meaning is then placed onto it.

However you choose to perform the following meditation, the most crucial step is to simply allow yourself to be with what is. By no means do you have to accept it or even think fondly of it. We all know what it's like to be forced to like something we dislike.

The healing comes from simply stopping the resistance to what is, quieting the mind, and allowing what will arise to arise.

If worries, thoughts, and fears enter your mind, tell them that you're going to put them off to the side just for the next ten minutes. After this meditation, if you want, you're welcome to pick them back up.

This meditation could be performed while lying on your back or sitting in a chair.

Meditation Exercise:

The Pain Body

1. Breath in deeply to the count of 3 and breath out to the count of 5. Repeat this three times.

2. Bring your attention from the outer world to the world inside of yourself. Connect with what it is you are feeling.

3. Pick an area of the pain or discomfort in your body to focus upon. If you'd like, you can lay your hands softly upon this region.

4. Ask yourself the following questions:

    *   What is the size of the pain or discomfort?

    *   The shape of it?

    *   The color of it?

    *   The intensity?

    *   The thickness?

    *   Is it moving or static?

5. Follow your pain for a moment. Notice how the sensation moves and changes when you focus on the subtlety.

    *   Has it changed since you started looking at it?

    *   What does it look like now?

6. Stay with the noticing. Allow the organic rise and fall of just what is to occur. Take a few moments to continue following the sensations. Notice how they morph and change. It is a universal law that nothing remains constant. Everything must change.

7. Begin to engage with this area as if it were a separate self. Ask it the following question:

   • Who are you?

   • What do you want me to know?

   Take time to allow it to fully express itself.

8. Check in with yourself as to how this part has shifted.

9. Make note of the wisdoms or insights the pain has provided you.

10. Thank these areas of your body for giving you relevant and useful information.

11. Before you end the meditation, create a picture in your mind of how you could take these newfound wisdoms and understandings with you as you continue with your day, all the way into the evening, to the moment you lay your head down and sleep peacefully throughout the night.

12. When you're ready, slowly begin to merge from the internal to the external. Notice the chair, bed or couch you are sitting or lying on. Wiggle your fingers and toes. As you open your eyes, notice the objects in the room, the clarity of your vision.

You are free now to continue on with your day.

Remember the wisdoms and messages from your body are always accessible and available to you, to guide you along your path towards a more positive, happier, and self aware you. All you need to do is slow down, quiet the mind, and listen.

15

Easing Pain Quick Reference

Use this table as a quick guide to assist you in targeting solutions to easing pain in your body. The left hand column lists areas where pain may occur. This second and third column describes postural factors and environmental causes that can contribute to different kinds of pain. The right-most column provides thumbnail solutions to easing the pain.

PAIN SITE	POSTURAL FACTORS	ENVIRONMENTAL CAUSES	SOLUTIONS
Carpal tunnel (tingling, burning, or numbness on the palm side of your first three and half fingers)	-Non neutral wrist postures (hyper flexion or extension) -A double whammy when typing too hard and with non-neutral finger posture -Pressure mid-wrist -Shoulders raised, rounded, and scrunched forward -Perched forward with head leaning forward -Neck side flexion	-Resting wrist on hard surface -Keyboard too high -Typing/mousing with wrist planted on table or wrist rest with wrist/hand extended back -Chair too low -Insufficient lumbar support -Monitor too far away -Chair too far away -Vibration -Hand utensils or tools too small -Pregnancy, gout or other conditions which cause the body to swell	-Float your wrists slightly above keyboard when typing -Incorporate gel wrist rests -Scoot back in your chair so your lumbar spine is properly supported -Scoot chair in close to your work station, then position the monitor at your optimal viewing distance -Neutral wrist! Consider using a wrist brace or elastic taping for positioning -Maintain the neutral "C" shape of your fingers when typing -Place a piece of standard tape on the back of your wrist in line with the third finger. This will provide you with feedback as to when the wrist is out of its neutral position -Lower the height of your keyboard to approximately belly button height or 2 inches below your elbow. (If you are a "hunt and peck" typist, the keyboard can be level with your elbow) -Consider a pullout keyboard platform tray -Raise height of chair so hips are just slightly higher than the knees -Consider anti-vibratory devices and tools -Consider building up handles, pens, and tools with foam or the like to widen and soften grip

PAIN SITE	POSTURAL FACTORS	ENVIRONMENTAL CAUSES	SOLUTIONS
Lower or mid-back pain	-Bending, twisting, or reaching without proper body mechanics -Perched forward in chair -Head/neck leaning forward of pelvis -Slouching in chair -Standing with knees locked and trunk and upper body overly rigid or slouched -Toes pointed outwards during standing or walking (external rotation) -Sitting with more pressure placed over one side of your pelvis than the other (i.e. when sitting with legs crossed)	-Chair too far away -Monitor too far away -Chair pulled back too far from work station -Insufficient lumbar support -Chair too low -Seat pan too short or too long -Frequently used items (filing cabinets, phones, customer service window off to one side) -Long periods of standing in one position, especially while looking down -Long periods of sustained and/or rigid static sitting without movement breaks -Frequent bending and/or looking down for items that are too low. Scanning items, laptop keyboard,or desktop items being too low -Heavy lifting with poor body mechanics -Unbalanced sitting and standing -Stress, tension, holding around low back/buttocks region -In rare cases, pain may be caused by other problems, such as gallbladder disease, cancer, or an infection	-Scoot all the way back into your chair so the back of your pelvis hits the back of the chair, and then slide the chair in towards the desk. Then, reposition the monitor for optimal viewing distance. -Adjust lumbar support to fit the small of your back -Keep your head positioned over your pelvis (head over tail) -If your chair lacks sufficient lumbar support, use a towel roll or external lumbar support -Adjust height of the chair so your hips are above your knees -Reposition your seat pan so there is 2-4 fingers behind your knees -Position frequently used items in closer reach to avoid twisting, bending, and extended reaching -Turn your belly button and sternum to face your work area -Use a standing mat if you stand for long periods of time -Position one foot in front of the other for sustained standing, bending, or twisting -Avoid long periods of static sitting by stretching every 20-30 minutes -Perform frequent back bends and stretches -Shift your weight between your legs and pelvis when seated and standing

PAIN SITE	POSTURAL FACTORS	ENVIRONMENTAL CAUSES	SOLUTIONS
Upper back	-Head/neck shoulders rounded forward -Rounded upper back -Inferior border of shoulder blades winged off thorax -Sustained neck flexion (See section above for more)	-Perching forward in chair with forward lean or hunched over a computer screen and looking down for sustained periods -Chair too low -Monitor too far away or too low -Over reliant upon chair arm rests when typing -Keyboard too high -"Hunt and peck" typist or frequently looking down to view keys or monitor -Frequent forward reach towards service window, keyboard or mouse, etc. -Bifocals (See section above for more)	-Position self properly in chair as discussed in section above -Raise chair so your hips are slightly higher than your knees -Lower your keyboard so your wrists are slightly lower than your elbows if you are a touch typist -Consider a keyboard platform tray -Consider learning to touch type or memorizing keys -Maintain a neutral neck posture

PAIN SITE	POSTURAL FACTORS	ENVIRONMENTAL CAUSES	SOLUTIONS
Lateral epicondylitis (tennis elbow)	-Extended wrists postures -Working with arms extended far away from torso -Gripping too tightly -Longer than average arms, particularly the humerus or upper arms -Edema or any sort of inflammatory conditions can also contribute to pressure and constriction in the elbow region	-Excessive forward or upward reach especially when combined with activities which require twisting, turning, and dexterous movements of the hand -Vibration -Grip size too large or too small -Common activities include playing tennis, repetitive reaching for a door handle or construction tasks such as drilling. Desk or house work that requires extensive and repetitive arm reaching	-Neutral wrists -Work with your elbows close by your sides -Avoid repetitive twisting or turning motions of the hand/wrist -Move your body closer to work area to avoid excessive reaching -Cover vibrating tools with viscoelastic materials or use anti-vibration gloves or covers (i.e., steering wheel covers) -Soften your grip -If possible, adjust grip size of your tool or instrument -Use a power grip (suggested handles should be cylindrical or oval in cross sections) -Tennis elbow strap placed slightly below your elbow -Ice massage five minutes three times per day, particularly after activities

PAIN SITE	POSTURAL FACTORS	ENVIRONMENTAL CAUSES	SOLUTIONS
Finger tingling in one finger only in a localized region	-Gripping too tightly -Statically holding one finger in extension while using the other fingers repetitively -Forceful use of fingers -Compression around finger	-Grip size too small -vibration and tight gripping of tool -Typing or mousing while habitually hyperextending the pinky and/or other fingers -Pounding keys while typing -Ring too tight	-Build up the grip size of tools -See tips for tool usage in section above -Purchase a larger and more contoured mouse, tape or place foam rubber padding around your pencil or pen or purchase a pen with a larger and softer grip -Maintain the "C" shape posture of your fingers when performing dexterous tasks such as typing and mousing -When reaching keys outside of the home row of your keyboard, move your entire hand rather than extending your fingers -Avoid repeated toggling with one hand -Type softer

PAIN SITE	POSTURAL FACTORS	ENVIRONMENTAL CAUSES	SOLUTIONS
Numbness tingling in elbow	- Leaning on elbow - Elbow bent, i.e fetal position when sleeping - Keyboard too high - Neck laterally flexed - Tense and raised shoulders/upper trapezium region - Edema or any sort of inflammatory conditions can contribute to pressure and constriction in the elbow region	- Sleep posture - Leaning on elbows when sitting for an extended period of time - Pressures on medial elbow - Cradling phone held between ear and shoulder	- Lower keyboard. Consider a keyboard platform if appropriate - Avoid putting pressure on elbow especially when typing. If you need to apply pressure, use a gel pad on edge of keyboard or apply padding to the surface top where contact is being made - If resting on armrest of chair, make sure there's sufficient padding and avoid any sharp edges. With arm rests, work surface height must be level or ever so slightly lower than your armrests - Sleep with your elbow straight rather than bent. Can put it in between two pillow cases in a pillow to prevent you from bending it at night

PAIN SITE	POSTURAL FACTORS	ENVIRONMENTAL CAUSES	SOLUTIONS
Tingling, burning, numbness in one or more fingers in inconsistent and spotty regions of your distal arms	-Head/neck shoulders rounded forward -Shoulders/upper trapezius raised -Tightness around your neck and jaw -Head/neck side bent -Wrist flexed and/or bent to side -Eye strain & anything that causes more tension around the head and face (i.e. stress) will also tighten the neck.	-Frequent head protruding or rounding forward or down or to the side to view monitor -Cradling the phone between your shoulder and neck -Arms raised too high to access your keyboard or desktop items -Working with your arms overhead -Sleeping with your head neck laterally flexed and/or slightly forward -Vibration &/or excess pressure in your hands	-Work with your shoulder's relaxed and lowered -Minimize overhead reaching; utilize a step stool -Reposition the monitor at the appropriate height and distance -Obtain a "hands free" headset for phone use -Work with your head/neck in neutral -Work with your wrist & arms in neutral. A wrist splint or taping can assist with this -Sleep with a neutral head/neck posture. Reposition or fit your pillow size accordingly -Soften your jaw and neck tension. Put a cork from a wine bottle into your mouth for a few minutes to break the "clenching" habit -Take more frequent vision and movement breaks -Perform the towel under neck ex. series

PAIN SITE	POSTURAL FACTORS	ENVIRONMENTAL CAUSES	SOLUTIONS
Shoulder/upper trapezium region	-Raised shoulders -Rounded hunched shoulders -Tightness around jaw and lower neck -Too much arm abduction	-Keyboard or work surface too high and/or far forward -Monitor too low or too far away -Mouse too far to the side of the keyboard -Chair too low -Armrests too high or low	-Lower keyboard or work surface (consider a keyboard platform tray) -Position the keyboard toward the front of your desk to avoid excessive forward reach -Raise chair and if needed get a footrest -Scoot in closer to your work surface. Reposition the monitor at the appropriate distance -Bring mouse closer to the keyboard -Decrease the mouse pointer speed -Consider left-handed mousing if pain on the right side -Reposition the chair armrests to the height of your elbow -Soften your jaw and neck. Can use cork (as mentioned above) -Do shoulder relaxation exercises -Use a headset for your phone as opposed to cradling it with your neck and shoulder.

PAIN SITE	POSTURAL FACTORS	ENVIRONMENTAL CAUSES	SOLUTIONS
Thoracic Outlet	-Frequent head protruding or rounding forward or down to view monitor -Cradling the phone between your shoulder and neck -Arms raised too high to access your keyboard or desktop items. -Working with your arms overhead -Sleeping with your head neck laterally flexed and/or slightly forward, and your arms bent up to your chest - Jaw clenching	-Phone to ear as opposed to headset -Anything that is causing shoulder and neck to be closer towards one another, compressing the area between the anterior and medial scalene and the first rib, compressing the neuro-vascular bundle	-Work with your shoulder's relaxed and lowered -Minimize overhead reaching. Utilize a step stool -Work with your arms in neutral. Adjust the chair height and keyboard height accordingly -Reposition the monitor at the appropriate height and distance -Obtain a "hands free" headset for phone use -Work with your head/neck in neutral -Sleep with a neutral head/neck posture. Reposition or fit your pillow accordingly -Soften your jaw and neck. Put a cork from a wine bottle into your mouth for a few minutes to break the "clenching" habit

PAIN SITE	POSTURAL FACTORS	ENVIRONMENTAL CAUSES	SOLUTIONS
Pain on side of neck	-Head turned to the side when working -Shoulders raised up -Tight jaw - See factors listed under Thoracic Outlet	-Monitor to the side -Mouse and other frequently used items to the side	-Move monitor to the middle -Move the mouse (or any frequently used items) to the left. Can alternate between right- and left-sided mousing -Perform eye "square" exercise on side that the neck range of motion is more limited - See factors listed under Thoracic Outlet

Appendix

Workshops and Consultations

Shara Ogin offers private consultations as well as workshops, retreats, and wellness seminars. Many people find live-learning a more enjoyable and meaningful way to learn because it allows for a more kinesthetic or feeling experience.

Live-learning is essential to bridge the gap from the conceptual and intellectual processing of information to a more somatic experience. Long-term change can only occur when we bring new learning from our minds into our internal sensory world where the information becomes ingrained and sub-corticalized and new motor learning occurs.

During immersions into these sensory and group learning experiences, people are able to take time to explore, feel and relearn options for moving and functioning in the world. Spending too much time hovering over the computer narrows our perspectives, changes the shape and articulations of our bones, and disconnects us from our surroundings.

I believe health and pain issues must be healed from the root.

And I thank you for taking the time to make your body and your health a priority.

For information about seminars and sessions, or to ask questions or make comments, please email: sharaogin@gmail.com

Printed in Great Britain
by Amazon

66649304R00071